Rapid Geriatric Assessment

Editor

JOHN E. MORLEY

CLINICS IN GERIATRIC MEDICINE

www.geriatric.theclinics.com

August 2017 • Volume 33 • Number 3

ELSEVIER

1600 John F. Kennedy Boulevard • Suite 1800 • Philadelphia, Pennsylvania, 19103-2899

http://www.theclinics.com

CLINICS IN GERIATRIC MEDICINE Volume 33, Number 3
August 2017 ISSN 0749–0690, ISBN-13: 978-0-323-53231-0

Editor: Jessica McCool
Developmental Editor: Colleen Dietzler

Clinics in Geriatric Medicine (ISSN 0749-0690) is published quarterly by Elsevier Inc., 360 Park Avenue South, New York, NY 10010-1710. Months of issue are February, May, August, and November. Business and Editorial Offices: 1600 John F. Kennedy Blvd., Suite 1800, Philadelphia, PA 191023-2899. Periodicals postage paid at New York, NY, and additional mailing offices. Subscription prices are $273.00 per year (US individuals), $590.00 per year (US institutions), $100.00 per year (US student/resident), $381.00 per year (Canadian individuals), $748.00 per year (Canadian institutions), $195.00 per year (Canadian student/resident), $402.00 per year (international individuals), $748.00 per year (international institutions), and $195.00 per year (international student/resident). Foreign air speed delivery is included in all *Clinics* subscription prices. All prices are subject to change without notice. POSTMASTER: Send address changes to *Clinics in Geriatric Medicine,* Elsevier Health Sciences Division, Subscription Customer Service, 3251 Riverport Lane, Maryland Heights, MO 63043. **Telephone: 1-800-654-2452 (U.S. and Canada); 314-447-8871 (outside U.S. and Canada). Fax: 314-447-8029. E-mail:** journalscustomerservice-usa@elsevier. com **(for print support) or** journalsonlinesupport-usa@elsevier.com **(for online support).**

Reprints. For copies of 100 or more, of articles in this publication, please contact the Commercial Reprints Department, Elsevier Inc., 360 Park Avenue South, New York, New York 10010-1710. Tel.: 212-633-3874; Fax: 212-633-3820, E-mail: reprints@elsevier.com.

Clinics in Geriatric Medicine is covered in *MEDLINE/PubMed (Index Medicus), EMBASE/Excerpta Medica, Current Contents/Clinical Medicine (CC/CM), and the Cumulative Index to Nursing & Allied Health Literature.*

Contributors

EDITOR

JOHN E. MORLEY, MB, BCh
Dammert Professor of Gerontology, Director, Division of Geriatric Medicine, Saint Louis University School of Medicine, St Louis, Missouri

AUTHORS

DAVID BECK, MD
Associate Professor, Department of Psychiatry and Behavioral Neuroscience, Saint Louis University, St Louis, Missouri

RICCARDO CALVANI, PhD
Researcher, Department of Geriatrics, Neurosciences and Orthopedics, Center for Geriatric Medicine (CEMI), Institute of Internal Medicine and Geriatrics, Catholic University of the Sacred Heart, Rome, Italy

MATTEO CESARI, MD, PhD
Associate Professor, Gérontopôle, University Hospital of Toulouse, University of Toulouse III-Paul Sabatier, Toulouse, France

NATALIA DEL CAMPO, PhD
Gérontopôle, Centre of Exellence in Neurodegeneration, Centre Hospitalier Universitaire de Toulouse, Toulouse, France

JULIEN DELRIEU, MD
Gérontopôle, Centre Hospitalier Universitaire de Toulouse, Toulouse, France

GUSTAVO DUQUE, MD, PhD
Geriatrician, Department of Aged Care, Director, Australian Institute for Musculoskeletal Science (AIMSS), Centre for Health, Research and Education, Sunshine Hospital, Western Health, Department of Medicine-Western Precinct, Melbourne Medical School, The University of Melbourne, St Albans, Victoria, Australia

JOSEPH H. FLAHERTY, MD
Professor, Division of Geriatrics, Department of Internal Medicine, Saint Louis University, St Louis, Missouri

BERTRAND FOUGÈRE, MD, PhD
Gérontopôle, Centre Hospitalier Universitaire de Toulouse, Inserm UMR1027, Université de Toulouse III Paul Sabatier, Toulouse, France

GEORGE T. GROSSBERG, MD
Professor, Departments of Psychiatry & Behavioral Neuroscience, Internal Medicine, Dementia, Health Aging and Anatomy & Neurobiology, Division of Geriatric Medicine, Saint Louis University, St Louis, Missouri

KAREEANN S.F. KHOW, MBChB, FRACP
Senior Clinical Lecturer and NHMRC PhD Candidate, Aged and Extended Care Services, The Queen Elizabeth Hospital, Central Adelaide Local Health Network and Adelaide Geriatrics Training and Research with Aged Care (GTRAC) Centre, School of Medicine, Faculty of Health and Medical Sciences, University of Adelaide, Woodville South, South Australia, Australia

FRANCESCO LANDI, MD, PhD
Department of Geriatrics, Neurosciences and Orthopedics, Center for Geriatric Medicine (CEMI), Institute of Internal Medicine and Geriatrics, Catholic University of the Sacred Heart, Rome, Italy

EMANUELE MARZETTI, MD, PhD
Assistant Professor, Department of Geriatrics, Neurosciences and Orthopedics, Center for Geriatric Medicine (CEMI), Institute of Internal Medicine and Geriatrics, Catholic University of the Sacred Heart, Rome, Italy

JOHN E. MORLEY, MB, BCh
Dammert Professor of Gerontology, Director, Division of Geriatric Medicine, Saint Louis University School of Medicine, St Louis, Missouri

ANNA PICCA, PhD
Department of Geriatrics, Neurosciences and Orthopedics, Center for Geriatric Medicine (CEMI), Institute of Internal Medicine and Geriatrics, Catholic University of the Sacred Heart, Rome, Italy

JAMES L. RUDOLPH, MD, SM
Associate Professor, Center of Innovation in Long Term Services and Support, Providence VAMC, School of Public Health, Brown School of Medicine, Providence, Rhode Island

ANGELA M. SANFORD, MD
Assistant Professor of Internal Medicine, Division of Geriatric Medicine, Saint Louis University School of Medicine, St Louis, Missouri

GAËLLE SORIANO
PhD Student, Gérontopôle, Centre Hospitalier Universitaire de Toulouse, Toulouse, France

SANDRINE SOURDET, MD
Gérontopôle, Centre Hospitalier Universitaire de Toulouse, Inserm UMR1027, Université de Toulouse III Paul Sabatier, Toulouse, France

DANIEL SWAGERTY, MD, MPH
Professor of Family Medicine and Internal Medicine, Associate Chair for Geriatrics and Palliative Care, Department of Family Medicine, Associate Director, Landan Center on Aging, University of Kansas School of Medicine, Kansas City, Kansas

BRUNO VELLAS, MD, PhD
Gérontopôle, Centre Hospitalier Universitaire de Toulouse, Inserm UMR1027, Université de Toulouse III Paul Sabatier, Toulouse, France

RENUKA VISVANATHAN, MBBS, FRACP, PhD
Clinical Director and Professor of Geriatric Medicine, Aged and Extended Care Services, The Queen Elizabeth Hospital, Central Adelaide Local Health Network and Adelaide Geriatrics Training and Research with Aged Care (GTRAC) Centre, School of Medicine, Faculty of Health and Medical Sciences, University of Adelaide, Woodville South, South Australia, Australia

JEAN WOO, MD
Department of Medicine and Therapeutics, Prince of Wales Hospital, The Chinese University of Hong Kong, Shatin, New Territories, Hong Kong

JIRONG YUE, MD
Professor, Department of Geriatrics, West China Hospital, Sichuan University, Chengdu, Sichuan, China

SYED NOMAN Y. ZAIDI, MD
Geriatric Psychiatry Resident, Department of Psychiatry and Behavioral Neuroscience, Saint Louis University, St Louis, Missouri

JESSE ZANKER, MBBS, BMedSci
Physician, Senior Research Fellow, Department of Aged Care, Sunshine Hospital, Western Health, St Albans, Victoria, Australia

Contents

Frailty is a clinical state characterized by a decrease of an individual's homeostatic reserves and is responsible for enhanced vulnerability to endogenous and/or exogenous stressors. Such a condition of extreme vulnerability exposes individuals to an increased risk of negative health-related outcomes. Multiple operational definitions of frailty are available in the literature, but none can be indicated as a gold standard. Frailty should be considered a condition of major interest for public health and become the lever for reshaping the obsolete health care systems currently unable to adequately address the clinical needs of aging populations.

Sarcopenia refers to age-related muscle loss, defined using a combination of appendicular muscle mass, muscle strength, and physical performance measures. The pathogenesis depends on a balance between positive and negative regulators of muscle growth. Sarcopenia increases the risk for falls, fractures, dependency, use of hospital services, institutionalization, poor quality of life, and mortality. In clinical practice, brief screening tools, such as the 5-item SARC-F score, may be useful. Although pharmacologic treatments are actively being studied, the current mainstay consists of optimizing nutrition status, in particular protein and vitamin D status, and resistance exercises.

Older people often experience loss of appetite and/or decreased food intake that, unavoidably, impact energy metabolism and overall health status. The association of age-related nutritional deficits with several adverse outcomes has led to the recognition of a geriatric condition referred to as "anorexia of aging." Anorexia is an independent predictor of morbidity and mortality both in the community and across clinical settings. Multidimensional interventions within personalized care plans currently represent the most effective option to ensure the provision of adequate amounts of food, limit weight loss, and prevent adverse health outcomes in older adults.

Mild cognitive impairment (MCI) occurs along a continuum from normal cognition to dementia. A roadblock to earlier diagnosis and potential treatment is the lack of consistency with screening for MCI. Universal screening would be ideal, but is limited. Once a diagnosis of MCI is made, it is important for the clinician to evaluate for reversible causes. At present time, there are no pharmacologic treatments proven to slow or cure progression of MCI to dementia; nonetheless, there is evidence that lifestyle modifications including diet, exercise, and cognitive stimulation may be effective.

Physical frailty is often associated with cognitive impairment, possibly because of common underlying pathophysiologic mechanisms. To stimulate research in this field, the concept *cognitive frailty* was proposed, emphasizing the important role of brain aging. Cognitive frailty was defined as the presence of cognitive deficits in physically frail older persons without dementia. This subtype of frailty is deemed important, as it may represent a prodromal phase for neurodegenerative diseases and is potentially a suitable target for early intervention. The aim of this report is to refine the framework for the definition and mechanisms of cognitive frailty and relevant screening tools.

The number of people living beyond 65 years of age is increasing rapidly, and they are at increased risk of falls. Falls-related injuries and hospitalizations are steadily increasing. Falls can lead to fear of falling, loss of independence, institutionalization, and death, inevitably posing a significant burden to the health care system. Therefore, screening of people at risk of falls and comprehensive assessment of older people at high risk of falls are critical steps toward prevention. This review evaluates the current knowledge relating to falls, with particular focus on rapid screening, assessment, and strategies to prevent falls in the community.

A comprehensive geriatric assessment, combined with a battery of imaging and blood tests, should be able to identify those hip fracture patients who are at higher risk of short- and long-term complications. This comprehensive assessment should be followed by the implementation of a comprehensive multidimensional care plan aimed to prevent negative outcomes in the postoperative period (short and long term), thus assuring a safe and prompt functional recovery while also preventing future falls and fractures.

Depression is common in geriatric patients, especially in those with multiple comorbidities and polypharmacy. Depression in older adults is often underdiagnosed and undertreated. Initial screening for depression can easily be accomplished in the waiting room. Yet the clinical interview still remains the gold standard for diagnosing geriatric depression. Key components of the clinical interview are observant watching of the patient for the subtle signs of depression. Clinical interview should be done with sensitivity to the importance of privacy. Illicit substances and medical conditions may significantly contribute. Suicide assessment should be done in a step wise manner.

Delirium is an acute change in attention and awareness that preferentially occurs in older patients with acute illness. This review provides an overview for clinicians with descriptions of the presentations (phenotypes), consequences, diagnosis, and screening of delirium. In addition, this review provides guidance for the challenges posed by delirium in a health care system, including implementation of delirium programs, tools to address the diagnosis and differential diagnosis of delirium, and a review of preventive and treatment studies with a goal of improving clinical practice.

This article provides an overview of how integrating quality palliative and end-of-life care into geriatric assessment can be a tremendous benefit to older adult patients and their families. Although the quality of palliative and end-of-life care for older adults has improved greatly, there are still many opportunities to improve the quality of life and function for older adult patients in the last few years of their life. More clinical expertise in comprehensive palliative and end-of-life care must be developed and maintained. There also must be greater focus and more direct reimbursement developed for physicians and health system providers.

The Rapid Geriatric Assessment (RGA) measures frailty, sarcopenia, anorexia, cognition, and advanced directives. The RGA is a screen for primary care physicians to be able to detect geriatric syndromes. Early intervention when geriatric syndromes are recognized can decrease disability, hospitalization, and mortality.

CLINICS IN GERIATRIC MEDICINE

THE CLINICS ARE AVAILABLE ONLINE!
Access your subscription at:
www.theclinics.com

Preface

The New Geriatric Giants

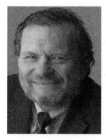

John E. Morley, MB, BCh
Editor

In 1965, Bernard Isaacs coined the term "geriatric giants." At that time, he named the geriatric giants as immobility, instability, incontinence, and impaired intellect/memory.[1] Over the subsequent fifty years, geriatrics has evolved, and today, the understanding of the modern "geriatric giants" has evolved to encompass the four new syndromes of frailty,[2] sarcopenia,[3] the anorexia of aging,[4] and cognitive impairment.[5] These conditions are the harbingers of falls,[6] hip fractures,[7] depression,[8] and delirium.[9] In this issue of the *Clinics in Geriatric Medicine*, we discuss in detail these "modern giants of geriatrics" and how early detection of these syndromes and intervention to correct these early signs of accelerated aging can reduce disability, hospitalization, institutionalization, and mortality.[10]

John E. Morley, MB, BCh
Division of Geriatric Medicine
Saint Louis University School of Medicine
1402 South Grand Boulevard, Room M238
St Louis, MO 63104, USA

E-mail address:
morley@slu.edu

REFERENCES

1. Morley JE. A brief history of geriatrics. J Gerontol A Biol Sci Med Sci 2004;59: 1132–52.
2. Morley JE, von Haehling S, Anker SD, et al. From sarcopenia to frailty: a road less traveled. J Cachexia Sarcopenia Muscle 2014;5:5–8.
3. Argiles JM, Muscaritoli M. The three faces of sarcopenia. J Am Med Dir Assoc 2016;17:471–2.
4. Morley JE. Pathophysiology of the anorexia of aging. Curr Opin Clin Nutr Metab Care 2013;16:27–32.

Clin Geriatr Med 33 (2017) xi–xii
http://dx.doi.org/10.1016/j.cger.2017.05.001
0749-0690/17/© 2017 Published by Elsevier Inc.

geriatric.theclinics.com

5. Morley JE, Morris JC, Berg-Weger M, et al. Brain health: the importance of recognizing cognitive impairment: an IAGG consensus conference. J Am Med Dir Assoc 2015;16:731–9.
6. Morley JE. Is it possible to prevent injurious falls? Eur Geriatr Med 2014;5:75–7.
7. Wendt K, Heim D, Josten C, et al. Recommendations on hip fractures. Eur J Trauma Emerg Surg 2016;42(4):425–31.
8. Gebretsadik M, Jayaprabhu S, Grossberg GT. Mood disorders in the elderly. Med Clin North Am 2006;90:789–805.
9. Rudolph JL. Arousal, attention, and an abundance of opportunity to advance delirium care. J Am Med Dir Assoc 2016;17(9):775–6.
10. Morley JE, Adams EV. Rapid geriatric assessment. J Am Med Dir Assoc 2015;16: 808–12.

Frailty in Older Persons

Matteo Cesari, MD, PhD[a],*, Riccardo Calvani, PhD[b],
Emanuele Marzetti, MD, PhD[b]

KEYWORDS

- Disability • Geriatrics • Assessment • Elderly • Prevention

KEY POINTS

- *Frailty* is defined as a clinical state characterized by an increased vulnerability of an organism to stressors, exposing individuals to negative health-related outcomes.
- Multiple operational definitions are available for capturing the risk profile of frail elders, but a gold standard is currently missing.
- The identification of frailty should lead to a comprehensive geriatric assessment (CGA) and personalized plan of intervention.
- Multidomain interventions are needed against frailty, but actions should be prioritized and carefully chosen to avoid overtreatment and adverse events.
- Novel models of care might be built up around the frailty condition to address the currently unmet clinical needs of older persons.

INTRODUCTION

The number of scientific publications on frailty has been increasing exponentially during the past 15 years (**Fig. 1**). Studies on the topic are not limited to the geriatric and gerontology fields, but discussions about frailty have also started appearing in other specialties and disciplines. Such a growing interest probably finds its common denominator in the severe burden that global aging is posing to society and public health systems.

The absolute and relative increase of older persons is a phenomenon occurring worldwide, from the richest to the poorest regions of the earth. At the same time, advanced age brings a higher likelihood of presenting multiple (often chronic and interacting) conditions, accentuated by frequent socioeconomic issues. The resulting scenario is characterized by a growing demand of care services for clinically complex elders, a population for which the application of standard decisional algorithms and

Disclosure Statement: The authors have nothing to disclose.
[a] Gérontopôle, University Hospital of Toulouse, University of Toulouse III-Paul Sabatier, 37 Allées Jules Guesde, Toulouse 31000, France; [b] Centro Medicina dell'Invecchiamento, Catholic University of the Sacred Heart, Largo Francesco Vito 1, Rome 00168, Italy
* Corresponding author.
E-mail address: macesari@gmail.com

Clin Geriatr Med 33 (2017) 293–303
http://dx.doi.org/10.1016/j.cger.2017.02.002
0749-0690/17/© 2017 Elsevier Inc. All rights reserved.
geriatric.theclinics.com

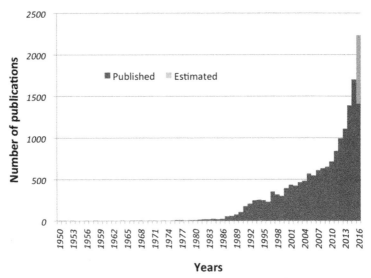

Years

Fig. 1. Number of scientific publications per year on frailty indexed in PubMed. Research updated on August 18, 2016, and conducted for the terms, "Frailty" and "Frail". (*Dark gray*) indexed articles; (*light gray*) estimated articles to be published from August 18, 2016, to the end of the year.

evidence is frequently challenging (due to the long-lasting and still detrimental evidence-based issue in geriatrics[1]).[2]

The concept of *frailty* can be found in the geriatric medicine literature in articles that first appeared in the 1950s and 1960s[3,4] and a more relevant body of contributions in the 1980s and 1990s (see **Fig. 1**). The condition of extreme vulnerability has always characterized the typical geriatric patient.[5] A more consistent and frequent use of the term frailty started, however, after the publication of its formal operational definitions. This is, although the birth of frailty is usually dated to 2001 (when the frailty phenotype was proposed by Fried and colleagues[6]), this condition had been object of study by geriatricians and gerontologists for several decades prior.

WHAT FRAILTY IS

Frailty is defined as a clinical state in which there is an increase in an individual's vulnerability to developing negative health-related events (including disability, hospitalizations, institutionalizations, and death) when exposed to endogenous or exogenous stressors.[7] This means that the same stressor may cause different consequences when soliciting a frail individual (ie, severe and prolonged functional loss and higher likelihood of incomplete recovery) compared with a robust person (ie, prompt and complete recovery with minor—if any—consequences).[8]

In parallel with the concept of frailty, the term, *resilience*, has started being used more frequently during the last few years. It is described as "the human ability to adapt in the face of tragedy, trauma, adversity, hardship, and ongoing significant life stressors."[9] Resilience explains why 2 apparently similar frail persons may react differently to the same negative stimulus. The one able to better cope with the stressor is considered characterized by higher resilience, which is the external resources that an organism has available for counteracting the negative forces challenging its homeostasis (eg, more robust social network and higher economic status).

Recently, the *World Report on Ageing and Health* published by the World Health Organization[2] has introduced the concepts of intrinsic capacity (ie, the composite of all the physical and mental capacities of an individual) and functional ability (ie, the health-related attributes that enable people to be and to do what they have reason to value), both presenting solid foundations in the geriatric background of frailty. It was stated in the report:

> ...The definition of frailty remains contested, but it can be considered as a progressive age-related decline in physiological systems that results in decreased reserves of intrinsic capacity, which confers extreme vulnerability to stressors and increases the risk of a range of adverse health outcomes...

It might be possible to think of frailty as an individual's deficits that modify the intrinsic capacity and determine (together with environmental barriers) the deviation from the functional ability trajectory.

THE RELATIONSHIP BETWEEN FRAILTY AND DISABILITY

The relationship between frailty and disability is controversial. Some investigators tend to avoid such a strict, arbitrary categorization and do not exclude a priori the possibility that a disabled individual may also be frail. After all, capturing a gradient of risk is always possible, even among the sickest individuals, as far as adequate instruments and methodologies are applied. This is, for example, the case of the conceptualization of frailty elaborated by Rockwood and colleagues[10] and Mitniski and colleagues.[11] Another body of literature prefers framing frailty as a predisability condition.[12,13] Following this approach, frailty becomes of special interest as a target condition for preventive interventions against disability. This is a legitimate and valid use of the frailty concept. At the same time, the definition of frailty becomes more challenging because it implies the addition of a threshold (to differentiate it from disability) to an already debated definition.

In the absence of an agreed gold standard, there are no right or wrong answers to this issue. Making use of good sense, it is reasonable to state that frailty (or the increased vulnerability to stressors) can be detected and measured in every living organism. At the same time, the frailty condition can be identified and used in special settings and populations for special and sectorial purposes (eg, as a target condition for preventing a negative outcome as disability), provided that adequate adaptations to methodologies are implemented.

THE ASSESSMENT OF FRAILTY

More than 40 operational definitions of frailty have been proposed in the literature (and the number is continuously increasing).[14] Every instrument has been shown to possess a certain capacity of predicting negative outcomes in the elderly. Nevertheless, each tool tends to identify a specific population at risk of negative outcomes, and the agreement of results across instruments remains modest.[15,16]

The frailty phenotype is probably the most popular model for assessing the condition of interest.[17] It was originally operationalized using the Cardiovascular Health Study database, and validated showing its capacity to predict falls, hospitalizations, incident disability, and mortality.[6] It was conceived to capture a physical condition of risk and differentiated from comorbidity and disability (although overlapping among the 3 was possible).[18] The frailty phenotype is based on 5 predetermined criteria (ie, involuntary weight loss, exhaustion, muscle weakness, slow gait speed, and sedentary behavior). The number of positive criteria defines the individual as frail ($\geq$3), prefrail (1–2), and robust (none).[6] This instrument has played a major role in the diffusion of the concept of frailty in the literature, perhaps for its easy-to-understand profile. Although it is often indicated as the most commonly used definition of frailty, it is probably more correct to refer to it as a model. As recently reported by Theou and colleagues,[19] the original definition is rarely applied without adaptations to the available resources and the studied populations. As discussed previously, the modification of 1 or more items has the potential to change the final result of the test, having a negative impact on the comparability of findings across studies.

An alternative (potentially complementary) model is the one designed by Rockwood and colleagues[10] and Mitnitski and colleagues,[11] the so-called Frailty Index. The Frailty Index estimates the accumulation of deficits occurring with the aging process.[20] It is arithmetically defined as the ratio between the deficits (ie, signs, symptoms, diseases, and disabilities) presented by an individual and the total number of deficits considered in the evaluation. Accordingly, it is not important which items are considered for computing the score but rather their quantity.[17] In the Frailty Index, each item counts for $1/n$ (whereas n is the total number of items considered in the computation). This means that 1 item is not able to substantially modify the final score. At the same time, if an item is clinically relevant, it unlikely is present alone but simultaneously occurs with others. Differently from the frailty phenotype, the Frailty Index is based on the results of a previous comprehensive assessment of a person and objectivizes a status of biological aging.[17] Because the Frailty Index is not based on predetermined items, but is computed using a critical mass of comprehensive information, it is particularly suitable for (1) being retrospectively implemented in existing databases built up for other purposes and (2) promoting interdisciplinary analyses and comparisons.[21–23] The arithmetical model at the basis of the Frailty Index has also been applied to animal models (for promoting translational research on frailty)[24] and biochemical results (for potentially anticipating the detection of the fragilization process).[25] The Frailty Index follows different objectives from other tools assessing frailty. It cannot be used for screening purposes because it is based on the results of a comprehensive geriatric assessment. Other instruments are instead based on quick-to-assess signs/symptoms to detect individuals in need of secondary and more in-depth assessment. The Frailty Index comes at a later stage, once such a comprehensive evaluation conducted by the specialist is completed to provide an objective value to the burden of deficits affecting the person.[17]

Another approach to frailty deserving special attention is the biopsychosocial model proposed by Gobbens and colleagues[26,27] and operationalized with the Tilburg Frailty Indicator.[28] This model has been attracting increasing interest in the scientific community for expanding the domain of frailty beyond the physical and clinical domain, toward social sciences. This step for a more global appreciation of frailty might be considered necessary if the role played by the socioeconomic context in determining the vulnerability status of an older person is taken into account.

A strategy to identify individuals exposed at increased risk of negative outcomes is use of the FRAIL acronym (ie, Fatigue, Resistance, Ambulation, Illnesses, and Loss of weight) proposed[29] and validated by Morley and colleagues[30] (**Table 1**). This simple tool easily reminds clinicians of 5 key aspects for evaluating the frailty status and selects those candidates worthy of further investigation. FRAIL stems from the frailty phenotype, includes a variable of clinical complexity (ie, multimorbidity), and overcomes one of the major limitations of the model proposed by Fried and colleagues,[6] that is its feasibility in daily outpatient routine. Although apparently easy to conduct, the frailty phenotype as originally designed is time consuming (eg, for the assessment

Table 1 The FRAIL instrument	
Symptom/Sign	Assessment
Fatigue	Are you fatigued?
Resistance	Cannot walk up one flight of stairs?
Ambulation	Cannot walk one block?
Illnesses	Do you have more than 5 illnesses?
Loss of weight	Have you lost more than 5% of your weight in the last 6 mo?

The presence of 3 or more positive answers defines the status of frailty; 1 or 2 positive answers identify prefrailty; the absence of positive answers indicates robustness.

of the Minnesota Leisure Time Physical Activity questionnaire) and requires the availability of specific devices (ie, dynamometer).

Besides these instruments, several other tools are available in the literature for describing a gradient of risk in older persons. Some have specifically been designed to support large-scale surveys to identify at-risk individuals in the community (eg, the INTER-FRAIL instrument and[31] the 6-item Sherbrooke Postal Questionnaire[32]). Others (as also the frailty phenotype itself[6]) have been developed from secondary analyses conducted in epidemiologic cohort studies (eg, the 3 criteria identified in the Study of Osteoporotic Fractures[33] or the 5 items retrieved from the Survey of Health, Ageing and Retirement in Europe database[34]).

Physical performance measures (eg, gait speed[35,36] and the Short Physical Performance Battery[37,38]) may also serve for capturing the increased vulnerability of an individual to stressors. These tests were originally designed for assessing the physical domain of an older person, but it is acknowledged that they are able to robustly estimate an individual's biological age.[39]

As discussed previously, the list of instruments for detecting frailty might be long and their descriptions are not within the aims of the present article. Moreover, the clinical condition of frailty is often confused with the mere result of the tests.[5] Instruments are important (especially in geriatric medicine) for supporting clinical decisions but cannot replace clinical judgment, especially if an instrument is designed for screening (and not diagnostic) purposes. Frailty is not a disease but only the first step for the eventual initiation of a specific care process (ie, the CGA and design of a person-tailored geriatric intervention).

THE MANAGEMENT OF FRAILTY

In a recent document, entitled *Fit for Frailty*,[40] edited by the British Geriatrics Society, the focus is on the intervention plan and not particularly to the detection of frailty. Multiple instruments are recommended for screening frailty (eg, gait speed,[41] Timed Up and Go test,[42] and the PRISMA-7 questionnaire[43]). Such large indications might hamper the possibility of standardizing care (ie, different instruments = different risk profiles = different needs). However, authors give more emphasis to the process leading to the CGA and person-tailored plan of intervention than to the screening procedures. The fact that the screening/assessment instrument is secondary to the proposed model of care also meets the need of providing a sufficiently flexible structure to be applied in diverse settings and populations.

It is well established that a relatively large proportion of older persons presents unmet clinical needs. At the same time, clinical needs are different across populations, settings, and geographic regions. Current recommendations discourage the systematic screening of frailty in the general population for obvious cost-effectiveness limitations.[44] Thus, the implementation of frailty in the clinical care first requires a careful evaluation of public health priorities and available resources. Such considerations are crucial for guiding the development of the model for taking care of frail elders. It is for this reason that the model should not be based on specific instruments but on a common theoretic strategy applied in different ways according to resources and needs.[45] For example, a highly sensitive instrument (ie, capable of better identifying true positive individuals) may be preferred in settings with limited resources. Differently, a more specific tool (ie, more accurate at excluding true negative subjects) might be preferred when resources allow for a larger-scale evaluation of the population. According to the interventions planned after the detection of a case, the system should equip itself with the adequate tools and infrastructures for conducting the best-allowed and feasible clinical practice.

Once the causes responsible for a frailty condition are detected, the geriatric expertise should prioritize interventions, balancing pros and cons according to an individual's characteristics, needs, and resources. This practice is hard to standardize within rigid decisional algorithms due to the heterogeneous complexity of frail elders and the often scarce evidence available for the elderly. Moreover, older persons often present socioeconomic and environmental risk factors hampering the efficacy of interventions that are exclusively or too focused on single clinical findings and biological parameters. The assessment of a frail elder that does not take into account the living environment and social network may result in insufficient (if not detrimental) solutions.[46] For these reasons, geriatric medicine is probably closer to an art than a rigid scientific discipline.[47] This explains why the role of the geriatrician in the management of frailty is so important and should not be easily delegated.[5] A Cochrane review shows that the efficacy of the CGA is closely related to the presence of a geriatrician in the management of frail elders.[48]

If the concept of frailty is widely considered (and not restricted to the results of a single, potentially biasing instrument), it is evident how coordinated actions aimed at prioritizing and personalizing interventions are effective across different clinical settings in the prevention of negative health-related events in the elderly.[49–52] Recent evidence developed after the implementation of frailty operationalizations, however, seems less promising. Several studies (especially conducted in primary care) have suggested the lack of positive findings for multidisciplinary interventions against frailty in the prevention of negative outcomes. Such an apparent contradiction might be explained in 2 different ways:

1. It has consistently been shown that more beneficial results are obtained from geriatric interventions when these are directed toward the frailest individuals. Interventions against minimally meaningful risk profiles are unlikely to modify the health status of older persons (due to a ceiling effect), especially when testing hard outcomes, such as disability. At the same time, the need for anticipating the detection of frailty in the community and primary care has been frequently advocated. This is important for prevention in aging societies. The healthier status of this subgroup of elders, however, automatically increases the number of false-positive cases, consequently watering down the effects of interventions (even when these may be relevant in other settings and for more severe risk profiles).

2. A relevant body of literature (largely coming from a nongeriatric background) has started translating frailty with the sterile results of questionnaires or tools. The screening tests have been used to diagnose frailty, because this was a disease

to treat. Consequently, several researchers have proposed that clinical benefits could be obtained by targeting the defining criteria of frailty (usually aspecific signs and symptoms). Adding interventions for the multiple abnormalities detected by screening tools has been considered a good way to go for assuring a multidomain approach and a holistic vision of patients. This is false if not dangerous, potentially leading to overtreatment and/or mistreatment (for the patient) and increased costs (for the health care system). Geriatricians know that multidomain interventions might be effective only when coordinated by a wise choice and prioritization of the solutions to implement.

Finally, it is important to discuss how the geriatric background and frailty experience may be implemented for individuals who are not chronologically old (as traditionally done up to date) but expressing typical geriatric conditions as a consequence of accelerated and/or accentuated aging (eg, individuals with Down syndrome[53,54] or other progeroid syndromes and patients with HIV infection[55,56]). For these individuals, most of the traditional frailty assessment tools are inadequate because they are designed and calibrated for elders. The defining items might not be easy to apply and/or the critical cutpoints may be inadequate. Again, instruments show how irrelevant they are in the face of the complexity of frailty and the importance of targeting this condition with person-tailored geriatric interventions.

SPECIFIC ISSUES IN THE MANAGEMENT OF FRAILTY

Interventions against frailty for preventing negative health-related outcomes are often justified by the expected benefits an individual may receive from earlier detection of unknown conditions. The anticipation of diagnoses may potentially provide the possibility of action when pathologic findings are still treatable and amenable to be reversed. Nevertheless, preventive strategies (especially when directed toward frail elders) imply special considerations involving ethical, clinical, and methodological issues.[57]

Looking for frailty means that a positive screening leads to further testing and examinations. This is legitimate and important, independently of a subject's age. In geriatric medicine, however, there is always the risk that a screening conducted for preventive purposes may open a Pandora's box without providing relevant health benefits for an individual. Defining a person as frail may lead to stigmatization and create a "patient" from a "relatively healthy" individual. The improvement of diagnostic techniques allows finding subtle but clinically meaningless abnormalities. Such abnormalities of uncertain relevance are responsible for overdiagnosis and overtreatment. In other and plainer words, the more that is looked for, the more is found. This same issue is currently under debate in fields where prevention has traditionally been considered crucial, such as oncology.[58,59] At the same time, prevention strategies are not free but instead are characterized by relevant costs for public health systems. Allocating money in the prevention may potentially imply a redistribution of public health budgets, reducing resources devoted to other care services. It is thus obvious that long-term investment in prevention is justifiable only when necessary and solidly proved. Therefore, the design of preventive strategies against frailty (especially in the nonclinical population) should well define a priori the target population according to the risk profile that has been shown to best respond to the planned interventions.

Last but not least, several studies have reported the possibility that frailty may spontaneously reverse. Accordingly, the positive results of a screening may become negative without the need of a specific intervention. Such fluctuations are part of the physiologic nature of the frailty condition, which does not follow a linear and easily

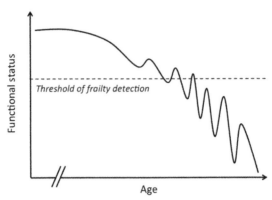

Fig. 2. Natural course of the frailty conditions characterized by more or less spontaneous fluctuations across the threshold of its detection.

predictable trajectory. The spontaneous modifications of frailty status over time are more likely to occur at the earliest and mildest stages of the disabling cascade (**Fig. 2**). Such a characteristic of frailty should raise cautiousness in screening of this condition, which potentially leads to treatment of nonclinically relevant and spontaneously reversible abnormalities. It should be stressed how the implementation of useless interventions not only is a waste of money and time but also may expose individuals (especially if in advanced age) to the risk of adverse events.

SUMMARY

Frailty is a geriatric condition of extreme relevance in aging societies. Frailty should become the lever for reshaping obsolete health care systems to make them more responsive to the needs of the aging populations. Frailty may be used to replace the old-fashioned criterion of chronologic age for defining a person as of geriatric interest. This can be done only if the identification of this risk profile is contextualized in systems through an adaptation of clinical approach, services, and care. For this purpose, the background and expertise gained by geriatricians over the years represent a useful resource. The integration of such knowledge of older persons in other disciplines and specialties for better addressing unmet clinical needs of frail individuals should be promoted. Models of interdisciplinary care for the management of geriatric patients (eg, orthogeriatric units[60,61]) suggest promising solutions.

REFERENCES

1. Cherubini A, Signore SD, Ouslander J, et al. Fighting against age discrimination in clinical trials. J Am Geriatr Soc 2010;58(9):1791–6.
2. World report on ageing and health. Geneva (Switzerland): World Health Organization; 2015.
3. Parfentjev IA. Frailty of old age and bacterial allergy. Geriatrics 1956;11(6):260–2.
4. Old and frail. Br Med J 1968;1(5594):723–4.
5. Cesari M, Marzetti E, Thiem U, et al. The geriatric management of frailty as paradigm of "The end of the disease era". Eur J Intern Med 2016;31:11–4.
6. Fried LP, Tangen CM, Walston J, et al. Frailty in older adults: evidence for a phenotype. J Gerontol A Biol Sci Med Sci 2001;56(3):M146–56.

7. Morley JE, Vellas B, Abellan van Kan G, et al. Frailty consensus: a call to action. J Am Med Dir Assoc 2013;14(6):392–7.

8. Clegg A, Young J, Iliffe S, et al. Frailty in elderly people. Lancet 2013;381:752–62.

9. Conti AA, Conti A. Frailty and resilience from physics to medicine. Med Hypotheses 2010;74(6):1090.

10. Rockwood K, Song X, MacKnight C, et al. A global clinical measure of fitness and frailty in elderly people. CMAJ 2005;173(5):489–95.

11. Mitnitski AB, Mogilner AJ, Rockwood K. Accumulation of deficits as a proxy measure of aging. ScientificWorldJournal 2001;1:323–36.

12. De Lepeleire J, Iliffe S, Mann E, et al. Frailty: an emerging concept for general practice. Br J Gen Pract 2009;59(562):e177–82.

13. Vellas B, Cestac P, Morley JE. Implementing frailty into clinical practice: we cannot wait. J Nutr Health Aging 2012;16(7):599–600.

14. Theou O, Walston J, Rockwood K. Operationalizing frailty using the frailty phenotype and deficit accumulation approaches. Interdiscip Top Gerontol Geriatr 2015; 41:66–73.

15. Hoogendijk EO, van der Horst HE, Deeg DJ, et al. The identification of frail older adults in primary care: comparing the accuracy of five simple instruments. Age Ageing 2013;42(2):262–5.

16. Theou O, Brothers TD, Mitnitski A, et al. Operationalization of frailty using eight commonly used scales and comparison of their ability to predict all-cause mortality. J Am Geriatr Soc 2013;61(9):1537–51.

17. Cesari M, Gambassi G, Abellan van Kan G, et al. The frailty phenotype and the frailty index: different instruments for different purposes. Age Ageing 2014; 43(1):10–2.

18. Fried LP, Ferrucci L, Darer J, et al. Untangling the concepts of disability, frailty, and comorbidity: implications for improved targeting and care. J Gerontol A Biol Sci Med Sci 2004;59(3):255–63.

19. Theou O, Cann L, Blodgett J, et al. Modifications to the frailty phenotype criteria: systematic review of the current literature and investigation of 262 frailty phenotypes in the Survey of Health, Ageing, and Retirement in Europe. Ageing Res Rev 2015;21:78–94.

20. Rockwood K, Mitnitski A. How might deficit accumulation give rise to frailty? J Frailty Aging 2012;1(1):8–12.

21. Guaraldi G, Brothers TD, Zona S, et al. A frailty index predicts survival and incident multimorbidity independent of markers of HIV disease severity. AIDS 2015; 29(13):1633–41.

22. Cesari M, Costa N, Hoogendijk EO, et al. How the frailty index may support the allocation of health care resources: an example from the INCUR study. J Am Med Dir Assoc 2016;17(5):448–50.

23. Kelaiditi E, Canevelli M, Andrieu S, et al. Frailty index and cognitive decline in Alzheimer's Disease: data from the impact of cholinergic treatment use study. J Am Geriatr Soc 2016;64(6):1165–70.

24. Feridooni HA, Sun MH, Rockwood K, et al. Reliability of a frailty index based on the clinical assessment of health deficits in male C57BL/6J mice. J Gerontol A Biol Sci Med Sci 2015;70(6):686–93.

25. Mitnitski A, Collerton J, Martin-Ruiz C, et al. Age-related frailty and its association with biological markers of ageing. BMC Med 2015;13:161.

26. Gobbens RJ, Luijkx KG, Wijnen-Sponselee MT, et al. In search of an integral conceptual definition of frailty: opinions of experts. J Am Med Dir Assoc 2010;11(5): 338–43.

27. Gobbens RJ, van Assen MA, Luijkx KG, et al. Testing an integral conceptual model of frailty. J Adv Nurs 2012;68(9):2047–60.

28. Gobbens RJ, van Assen MA, Luijkx KG, et al. The tilburg frailty indicator: psychometric properties. J Am Med Dir Assoc 2010;11(5):344–55.

29. Morley JE. Frailty: a time for action. Eur Geriatr Med 2013;4:215–6.

30. Morley JE, Malmstrom TK, Miller DK. A simple frailty questionnaire (FRAIL) predicts outcomes in middle aged African Americans. J Nutr Health Aging 2012; 16(7):601–8.

31. Mossello E, Profili F, Di Bari M, et al. Postal screening can identify frailty and predict poor outcomes in older adults: longitudinal data from INTER-FRAIL study. Age Ageing 2016;45(4):469–74.

32. Hebert R, Bravo G, Korner-Bitensky N, et al. Predictive validity of a postal questionnaire for screening community-dwelling elderly individuals at risk of functional decline. Age Ageing 1996;25(2):159–67.

33. Ensrud K, Ewing SK, Taylor BC, et al. Comparison of 2 frailty indexes for prediction of falls, disability, fractures, and death in older women. Arch Intern Med 2008; 168(4):382–9.

34. Romero-Ortuno R, Walsh CD, Lawlor BA, et al. A frailty instrument for primary care: findings from the Survey of Health, Ageing and Retirement in Europe (SHARE). BMC Geriatr 2010;10:57.

35. Studenski S, Perera S, Patel K, et al. Gait speed and survival in older adults. JAMA 2011;305(1):50–8.

36. Studenski S, Perera S, Wallace D, et al. Physical performance measures in the clinical setting. J Am Geriatr Soc 2003;51(3):314–22.

37. Guralnik JM, Simonsick EM, Ferrucci L, et al. A short physical performance battery assessing lower extremity function: association with self-reported disability and prediction of mortality and nursing home admission. J Gerontol 1994; 49(2):M85–94.

38. Guralnik JM, Ferrucci L, Simonsick EM, et al. Lower-extremity function in persons over the age of 70 years as a predictor of subsequent disability. N Engl J Med 1995;332(9):556–61.

39. Cesari M. Role of gait speed in the assessment of older patients. JAMA 2011; 305(1):93–4.

40. Fit for Frailty - consensus best practice guidance for the care of older people living in community and outpatient settings - a report from the British Geriatrics Society. British Geriatrics Society; 2014.

41. Abellan van Kan G, Rolland YM, Andrieu S, et al. Gait speed at usual pace as a predictor of adverse outcomes in community-dwelling older people an International Academy on Nutrition and Aging (IANA) Task Force. J Nutr Health Aging 2009;13(10):881–9.

42. Podsiadlo D, Richardson S. The timed "Up & Go": a test of basic functional mobility for frail elderly persons. J Am Geriatr Soc 1991;39(2):142–8.

43. Hébert R, Durand PJ, Dubuc N, et al, PRISMA Group. Frail elderly patients. new model for integrated service delivery. Can Fam Physician 2003;49:992–7.

44. Turner G, Clegg A. Best practice guidelines for the management of frailty: a British Geriatrics Society, age UK and Royal College of general practitioners report. Age Ageing 2014;43(6):744–7.

45. Cesari M, Prince M, Thiyagarajan JA, et al. Frailty: an emerging public health priority. J Am Med Dir Assoc 2016;17(3):188–92.

46. Marzetti E, Sanna T, Calvani R, et al. Brand new medicine for an older society. J Am Med Dir Assoc 2016;17(6):558–9.

47. Hadley EC. The science of the art of geriatric medicine. JAMA 1995;273(17): 1381–3.
48. Ellis G, Whitehead MA, O'Neill D, et al. Comprehensive geriatric assessment for older adults admitted to hospital. Cochrane Database Syst Rev 2011;(7):CD006211.
49. Stuck AE, Aronow HU, Steiner A, et al. A trial of annual in-home comprehensive geriatric assessments for elderly people living in the community. N Engl J Med 1995;333(18):1184–9.
50. Stuck AE, Minder CE, Peter-Wüest I, et al. A randomized trial of in-home visits for disability prevention in community-dwelling older people at low and high risk for nursing home admission. Arch Intern Med 2000;160(7):977–86.
51. Bernabei R, Landi F, Gambassi G, et al. Randomised trial of impact of model of integrated care and case management for older people living in the community. BMJ 1998;316(7141):1348–51.
52. Rubenstein LZ, Josephson KR, Wieland GD, et al. Effectiveness of a geriatric evaluation unit. A randomized clinical trial. N Engl J Med 1984;311(26):1664–70.
53. Carfi A, Antocicco M, Brandi V, et al. Characteristics of adults with down syndrome: prevalence of age-related conditions. Front Med (Lausanne) 2014;1:51.
54. Hermans H, Evenhuis HM. Multimorbidity in older adults with intellectual disabilities. Res Dev Disabil 2014;35(4):776–83.
55. Kooij KW, Wit FW, Schouten J, et al. HIV infection is independently associated with frailty in middle-aged HIV type 1-infected individuals compared with similar but uninfected controls. AIDS 2016;30(2):241–50.
56. Pathai S, Bajillan H, Landay AL, et al. Is HIV a model of accelerated or accentuated aging? J Gerontol A Biol Sci Med Sci 2014;69(7):833–42.
57. Cesari M, Vellas B. Frailty in clinical practice. Nestle Nutr Inst Workshop Ser 2015; 83:93–8.
58. Harding C, Pompei F, Burmistrov D, et al. Breast cancer screening, incidence, and mortality across US counties. JAMA Intern Med 2015;175(9):1483–9.
59. Howrey BT, Kuo YF, Lin YL, et al. The impact of PSA screening on prostate cancer mortality and overdiagnosis of prostate cancer in the United States. J Gerontol A Biol Sci Med Sci 2012;68(1):56–61.
60. Antonelli-Incalzi R, Gemma A, Capparella O. Orthogeriatric unit: a thinking process and a working model. Aging Clin Exp Res 2008;20(2):109–12.
61. Adunsky A, Lerner-Geva L, Blumstein T, et al. Improved survival of hip fracture patients treated within a comprehensive geriatric hip fracture unit, compared with standard of care treatment. J Am Med Dir Assoc 2011;12(6):439–44.

Sarcopenia

Jean Woo, MD

KEYWORDS

- Sarcopenia • Muscle mass • Sarcopenic obesity • Myostatin • Exercise
- Selective androgen receptor agonist

KEY POINTS

- Sarcopenia represents loss of muscle mass with age, and is defined by using measures of mass, strength, and physical functional performance.
- Muscle mass and function are affected by genetic, physiologic, and environmental factors, and are dependent on a dynamic balance between positive and negative regulators of muscle growth.
- Sarcopenia is a risk factor for falls, fractures, disability, dependency, poor quality of life, increased use of hospital services, institutionalization, and mortality.
- Raid screening tools, such as the SARC-F, are useful in the clinical setting to inform management.
- Treatment is mainly nonpharmacological (resistance exercise and optimizing nutrition, especially protein and vitamin D); various drugs are being developed but are largely undergoing phase 1 or 2 trials.

INTRODUCTION

Sarcopenia is a term first coined by Rosenberg in 1989[1] to draw attention to the age-related loss of muscle mass, with aging as a geriatric syndrome with adverse consequences that may be amenable to prevention and treatment. Although decline of muscle mass had been documented as a physiologic phenomenon, being approximately 8% per decade between 50 and 70 years, with the rate of decline accelerating to between 10% and 15% per decade after 70 years,[2] initially there was debate about whether sarcopenia was a disease or a natural phenomenon. After 2 to 3 decades of explosive research and publications in this area, the current consensus is that it is a condition that can be diagnosed, the presence of which leads to many adverse health outcomes that are common among older people, and that it may be prevented or managed by nonpharmacologic as well as pharmacologic means. This article describes the definition, prevalence, etiology, consequences, relationship with other syndromes and diseases, diagnosis, and treatment.

Disclosure Statement: The author has nothing to disclose.
Department of Medicine and Therapeutics, Prince of Wales Hospital, The Chinese University of Hong Kong, 9/F, Lui Che Woo Clinical Sciences Building, Shatin, New Territories, Hong Kong
E-mail address: jeanwoowong@cuhk.edu.hk

DEFINITION

Historically, sarcopenia was defined in terms of skeletal muscle mass adjusted only for height[3]; however, the current consensus includes measures of strength and physical performance. As there appear to be population variations in measures of muscle mass and strength, whether due to ethnic differences in body shape or sizes, or to environmental influences during the life course, definitions of sarcopenia vary with respect to cutoff values.[4,5] These definitions were determined from International Consensus Panels, with or without a data-driven approach deriving cutoff values from mobility limitation measures in large cohort studies (**Table 1**).[6-9]

PREVALENCE (REVERSIBILITY)

Prevalence of sarcopenia varies across geographic regions, age groups studied, and settings, from 1% to 29% in community-dwelling older people, 14% to 33% in long-term care, and 10% in acute hospital care populations.[7] Recently, it has been pointed out that sarcopenia is a condition that undergoes dynamic changes with time, in which improvement may be observed as well as decline.[10]

ETIOLOGY

Causes range from genetic, physiologic, and environmental factors. Studies on the molecular mechanisms in the pathogenesis of sarcopenia suggest that normal muscle mass and function are dependent on a dynamic balance between positive and negative regulators of muscle growth.[11] A shift of the balance toward negative regulators, likely resulting in expression of the C-terminal agrin fragment (indicating neuromuscular junction dysfunction) and skeletal muscle specific troponin T (sTnT), forms the main mechanism underlying sarcopenia (**Table 2**).

Age-related changes occur in muscle fiber structure and the neuromuscular junction, in muscle contractile properties as a result of muscle morphologic changes, neurodegenerative changes resulting in loss of muscle motor units, altered muscle protein metabolism, protein anabolic failure, hormone resistance syndromes, upregulation of inflammatory cytokines, oxidative damage affecting mitochondrial energy metabolism, poor nutritional status, and physical inactivity (**Figs. 1** and **2**).[12-21]

Nutritional factors and physical inactivity are major modifiable causes for sarcopenia. Reduction of food intake with aging is commonly observed[14] (also referred to as

Table 1
Comparison of different definitions of sarcopenia

Different Definitions	ASMI, kg		ASM/BMI, kg		GS, kg		WS, m/s	
	Men	Women	Men	Women	Men	Women	Men	Women
AWGS	<0.7	<5.4	—	—	<26	<18	<0.8	
EWGSOP	<6.52	<5.44	—	—	≤28	≤18	<0.8	
IWGS	≤7.23	≤5.67	—	—	—	—	<1	
FNIH	—	—	<0.789	<0.512	<26	<16	—	
FNIH Slowness	—	—	—	—	—	—	<0.8	

Abbreviations: ASM, appendicular skeletal mass; ASMI, appendicular skeletal mass index; AWGS, Asian Working Group on Sarcopenia; BMI, body mass index; EWGSOP, European Working Group on Sarcopenia in Older People; FNIH, Foundation of the National Institutes of Health; GS, grip strength; IWGS, International Working Group on Sarcopenia; WS, walking speed.

Table 2 Regulators of muscle mass and function	
Positive	**Negative**
• Bone morphogenic proteins (BMP)	• Transforming growth factor β (TGFβ)
• Brain-derived neurotrophic factor (BDNF)	• Myostatin
• Follistatin (FST)	• Activins A and B
• Irisin	• Growth and differentiating factor (GDF-15)

anorexia of aging), as a result of age-related changes in loss of appetite, sense of taste and smell, poor oral health, gastrointestinal changes (delay in gastric emptying and elevated cholecystokinin levels), dementia, depression, dependency, and social environment. Decline in neuropeptide Y (NPY) levels and function in the central nervous system and a decrease in nitric oxide activity is thought to play a key role in the anorexia of aging.[15] Decrease in calorie, and protein intake in particular, has adverse consequences for muscle health. Protein intake in excess of the amount to maintain nitrogen balance is thought to be required, from studies of protein intake and clinical studies of muscle mass and function, the recommendation being at least 1.2 g/kg of body weight.[16–19] Physical inactivity, such as bed rest during illness or habitually taking fewer steps, predisposes to loss of muscle strength and power. In healthy older adults, 10 days of bed rest results in loss of leg strength, power, and aerobic capacity.[20] Even a relative reduction in ambulation, measured as the number of steps taken each day, results in reduction in muscle mass and strength.[21]

CONSEQUENCES

Reduction in muscle mass has metabolic consequences, in increased insulin resistance and Vo$_2$ max, a measure of cardiorespiratory fitness. Decline in muscle mass, strength, and power also gives rise to various adverse consequences that reinforce each other in a downhill spiral toward poor quality of life, dependency, use of hospital services, institutionalization, and ultimately mortality. In a 4-year prospective study of community-dwelling older people in the United States, low thigh muscle cross-sectional area increased the risk of incident mobility limitations, activities of daily living, and incident fractures.[22,23] Other studies in Europe, the United States, and China showed that sarcopenia is a risk factor for falls,[24] fractures,[25,26] old age

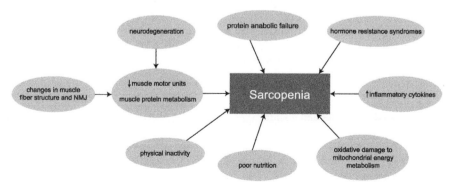

Fig. 1. Pathways leading to age-related decline in muscle mass and function. NMJ, neuromuscular junction.

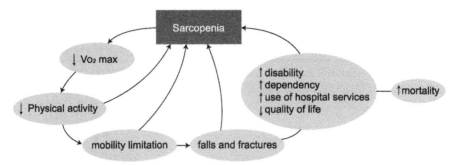

Fig. 2. Consequences.

disability,[27] impairment in activities of daily living,[28] development of disability,[29] and mortality.[30] A number of studies have reported on associations between the physical health component of the SF-36 quality-of-life instrument and sarcopenia.[28–30]

OTHER CLOSELY RELATED SYNDROMES AND DISEASES

Sarcopenic obesity (SO) is an emerging clinical entity characterized by excessive fat mass in the presence of reduced muscle mass. Although the term is predominantly used for older people, it also may be used in younger obese people on weight reduction programs or with chronic wasting diseases. The pathogenesis of SO is an additive component to sarcopenia through lipotoxicity on muscle, giving rise to muscle anabolic resistance (**Box 1**).[31] SO produces a double metabolic burden from low muscle mass, as well as excess adiposity, affecting cardio-metabolic and physical functions. There is no universal definition of SO, although many studies classify individuals with SO if they have appendicular mass fulfilling the criteria of sarcopenia in the presence of a body mass index in the obese category. A simple criterion of total body fat to leg muscle mass ratio has been proposed, and has shown to predict incident physical limitation in 3153 community-dwelling adults.[32] Another study used waist circumference as an indicator of central obesity and midarm muscle circumference as an indicator of sarcopenia, showing that men with SO had the highest all-cause mortality.[33]

Frailty, a geriatric syndrome that has emerged in the past 2 decades, is closely related to sarcopenia. Frailty describes a failure of the body to withstand external stressors, characterized by the phenotype of fatigue and slowness.[34] Another approach is characterization using the concept of multiple deficits.[35] Both frailty and sarcopenia have a similar impact on physical function and independence, and share common clinical features and underlying pathology, such as muscle weakness and poor physical performance measures, with upregulation of inflammatory cytokines. In parallel, research into diagnosis and treatment has increased as for sarcopenia,

---

Box 1
Closely related syndromes and diseases

- Sarcopenic obesity
- Frailty
- Cachexia and wasting disorders
- Sarco-osteoporosis

as described by Joseph H. Flaherty and colleagues in the article, "Dissecting Delirium: Phenotypes, Consequences, Screening, Diagnosis, Prevention, Treatment and Program Implementation," in this issue. Although sarcopenia is not specific to elderly individuals, and clinical features may overlap with cachexia and other wasting disorders, frailty may be considered a multidimensional geriatric syndrome, of which a physical aspect may include sarcopenia.

Muscle loss is also a prominent feature of cachexia that accompanies neoplastic and other chronic diseases, such as renal, cardiac, and pulmonary obstructive diseases. Cachexia is a complex metabolic syndrome that accompanies underlying life-limiting illnesses, with prominent weight loss and muscle wasting, with or without the loss of fat mass. It is not confined to elderly individuals; in children, it is manifested as failure to thrive. Although anorexia, inflammation, insulin resistance, and increased muscle protein breakdown are common features, inflammatory cytokines, such as tumor necrosis factor and interleukin-6, are highly elevated in cachexia compared with sarcopenia.[36]

The close relationship between muscle and bone has given rise to the term "sarco-osteoporosis." Both share common developmental origins, functional purpose, clinical associations, contribution to adverse health outcomes, such as fractures and disability, and have mutual influence on each other through myokines and osteokines. Homeostasis exists between muscle and bone via paracrine and mechanical factors, such that muscle and bone may be considered as one functional unit. Sarcopenia combined with use of the fracture prediction tool FRAX improves risk prediction in older men.[37] Strategies to prevent decline and maintenance of function, and nonpharmacologic as well as pharmacologic therapeutic strategies, may apply to both. For example, myostatin inhibitors increase both muscle force and bone density in mice.[38]

DIAGNOSIS

Diagnosis in the research setting tends to follow Consensus Panel and Foundation of the National Institutes of Health criteria listed previously, which involve measurements of grip strength, body composition using either dual-energy X-ray absorptiometry or bio-impedance, and physical performance measures. These diagnoses have been validated in prospective studies looking at incident mobility limitations or decline in physical performance measures.[9,39] However, such studies highlight the variability of absolute cutoff values in diagnosis, likely a consequence of ethnic and geographic variations in muscle mass, muscle strength, and physical performance measures.[4,40]

In the clinical setting, such diagnostic methods are difficult to incorporate because of time and resource limitations. At the same time, diagnosis is important, as measures should be implemented to prevent further functional decline or to achieve improvement in physical function. The 5-item questionnaire SARC-F has been compared with 3 consensus definitions from the United States, Europe, and Asia in a prospective study, in terms of predictive power for 4-year physical limitation and physical performance measures. The SARC-F has excellent specificity but poor sensitivity for sarcopenia classification, and is comparable to the other 3 methods.[9] The SARC-F has also been shown to have good internal consistency and validity in predicting mortality and health outcomes in 3 US longitudinal surveys: African American Health Study, Baltimore Longitudinal Study of Aging, and National Health and Nutrition Examination Survey.[41] Use of this tool could be the first step in community screening or in primary care practice, which could then be followed by more detailed resource-intensive assessments (**Table 3**).[42]

Table 3
SARC-F screen for sarcopenia

Component	Question	Scoring
Strength	How much difficulty do you have in lifting and carrying 10 pounds?	None = 0 Some = 1 A lot or unable = 2
Assistance in walking	How much difficulty do you have walking across a room?	None = 0 Some = 1 A lot, use aids, or unable = 2
Rise from a chair	How much difficulty do you have transferring from a chair or bed?	None = 0 Some = 1 A lot or unable without help = 2
Climb stairs	How much difficulty do you have climbing a flight of 10 stairs?	None = 0 Some = 1 A lot or unable = 2
Falls	How many times have you fallen in the past year?	None = 0 1–3 falls = 1 4 or more falls = 2

From Malmstrom TK, Morley JE. SARC-F: a simple questionnaire to rapidly diagnose sarcopenia. J Am Med Dir Assoc 2013;14:531; with permission.

TREATMENT (NONPHARMACEUTICAL AND PHARMACEUTICAL)
Nonpharmaceutical

Nutrition
For the management of sarcopenia, nutrition should be optimized by ensuring adequate amounts of macronutrients and micronutrients, summarized as follows: calories should be 24 to 36 kcal/kg per day; a minimum daily protein intake of 1.0 g/kg body weight, up to 1.5 g spread evenly over 3 meals; maintenance of serum vitamin D levels to 100 nmol/L (40 ng/mL) from vitamin D–rich diet or vitamin D supplementation. Supplementation with creatine monohydrate, antioxidants, amino acid metabolites, omega-3 fatty acids, and other compounds are actively being studied, with some promising results (**Box 2**).

A review on the effectiveness of nutrition supplementation on sarcopenia defined according to the European Working Group on Sarcopenia in Older People (EWGSOP) carried out by the International Sarcopenia Initiative in 2013,[7] identified 22 studies including dietary protein supplementation, amino acid supplements, and hydroxymethylbutyrate supplementation on muscle mass, muscle strength, and physical performance. These have variable beneficial effects on the 3 parameters, with or without exercise. Recently, leucine supplementation plus resistance training exercise showed increase in length strength and certain components of functional status.[43]

Exercise
Physical activity, in particular resistance training, is the cornerstone for increasing muscle strength and physical performance. The American College of Sport Medicine and American Heart Association recommend weight training 2 or 3 times a week to achieve gains in muscle size and strength, even in frail older persons.[44,45] Similar conclusions were drawn from a systematic review carried out by the International Sarcopenia Initiative in 2013.[7] Recent trials have examined multicomponent exercises consisting of muscle power combined with balance and gait training in frail nonagenarians, showing increase in cross-sectional muscle area, improved muscle strength and power, improved time up and go test with single and dual task, and balance.[46] The

---

Box 2
Nutritional recommendations

- Calories
- Proteins and amino acids
- Vitamin D
- Creatine monohydrate
- Antioxidants
- Amino acid metabolites and precursors betahydroxy
- Betamethylbutyrate and ornithine alpha ketoglutarate
- Omega-3 fatty acids
- Ursolic acid
- Nitrate and nitrate-rich foods
- Caloric restriction mimetics
- Exercise mimetics and gymnomimetics
- Manipulation of the gut microbiota

Data from Calvani R, Miccheli A, Landi F, et al. Current nutritional recommendations and novel dietary strategies to manage sarcopenia. J Frailty Aging 2013;2(1):38–53.

---

beneficial effects of exercise may be moderated by myostatin inhibition through increased hepatic synthesis of follistatin, a myostatin inhibitor, and also by stimulating anabolic hormone responses, including growth hormone and testosterone. It has been pointed out that such "exercise medicine" may have advantages of the single-drug approach in being more physiologic and free of side effects.[47] Currently, the strategy of combined nutrition supplementation and exercise appears to be the most promising one in the management of sarcopenia.

Pharmaceutical

Trials have been carried out for the drugs listed in **Box 3**.[48–50] However few have progressed to phase 3 or 4 clinical trials in older adults.

Box 3
Summary of drugs under trial

- Testosterone
- Selective androgen receptor agonists (SARMs)
- Growth hormone
- Insulinlike growth factor 1
- Ghrelin
- Leptin
- Vitamin D
- Myostatin inhibitor (REGN1033)
- Angiotensin-converting enzyme inhibitors
- Espindolol

Box 4
Biomarkers to monitor treatment

- Myostatin
- C-Terminal Agrin Fragment (CAF)
- Insulinlike growth factor 1
- Growth differentiation factor 15
- Activin A
- Follistatin
- Strength and power, per unit muscle mass

There are many regulatory requirements to be overcome in conducting such trials. There is a need for a universally agreed perspective that sarcopenia is a disease with a widely accepted diagnosis rather than a consequence of aging. Relevant primary and secondary outcomes need to be established. Functional outcome in terms of mobility limitation and/or physical performance measures seem to be widely accepted as the primary outcome together with muscle strength/power or mass. Biomarkers are increasingly being proposed to monitor treatment, even though there is no universal consensus (**Box 4**).[11,51]

REFERENCES

1. Rosenberg IH. Sarcopenia: origins and clinical relevance. J Nutr 1997;127(5 Suppl):990S–1S.
2. Grimby G, Saltin B. The ageing muscle. Clin Physiol 1983;3(3):209–18.
3. Baumgartner RN, Koehler KM, Gallagher D, et al. Epidemiology of sarcopenia among the elderly in New Mexico. Am J Epidemiol 1998;147(8):755–63 [Erratum appears in Am J Epidemiol 1999;149(12):1161].
4. Woo J, Arai H, Ng TP, et al. Ethnic and geographic variations in muscle mass, muscle strength and physical performance measures. Eur Geriatr Med 2014;5: 155–64.
5. Dodds RM, Syddall HE, Cooper R, et al. Global variation in grip strength: a systematic review and meta-analysis of normative data. Age Ageing 2016;45(2): 209–16.
6. Fielding RA, Vellas B, Evans WJ, et al. Sarcopenia: an undiagnosed condition in older adults. Current consensus definition: prevalence, etiology, and consequences. International Working Group on Sarcopenia. J Am Med Dir Assoc 2011;12(4):249–56.
7. Cruz-Jentoft AJ, Landi F, Schneider SM, et al. Prevalence of and interventions for sarcopenia in ageing adults: a systematic review. Report of the International Sarcopenia Initiative (EWGSOP and IWGS). Age Ageing 2014;43(6):748–59.
8. Chen LK, Liu LK, Woo J, et al. Sarcopenia in Asia: consensus report of the Asian Working Group for Sarcopenia. J Am Med Dir Assoc 2014;15(2):95–101.
9. Woo J, Leung J. Anthropometric cut points for definition of sarcopenia based on incident mobility and physical limitation in older Chinese people. J Gerontol A Biol Sci Med Sci 2016;71(7):935–40.
10. Yu R, Wong M, Leung J, et al. Incidence, reversibility, risk factors and the protective effect of high body mass index against sarcopenia in community-dwelling older Chinese adults. Geriatr Gerontol Int 2014;14(Suppl 1):15–28.

11. Kalinkovich A, Livshits G. Sarcopenia–the search for emerging biomarkers. Ageing Res Rev 2015;22:58–71.

12. Christensen K, McGue M, Yashin A, et al. Genetic and environmental influences on functional abilities in Danish twins aged 75 years and older. J Gerontol A Biol Sci Med Sci 2000;55(8):M446–52.

13. Lang T, Streeper T, Cawthon P, et al. Sarcopenia: etiology, clinical consequences, intervention, and assessment. Osteoporos Int 2010;21(4):543–59.

14. Bales CW, Ritchie CS. Sarcopenia, weight loss, and nutritional frailty in the elderly. Annu Rev Nutr 2002;22:309–23.

15. Morley JE, Farr SA. Cachexia and neuropeptide Y. Nutrition 2008;24(9):815–9.

16. Paddon-Jones D, Rasmussen BB. Dietary protein recommendations and the prevention of sarcopenia. Curr Opin Clin Nutr Metab Care 2009;12(1):86–90.

17. Volkert D, Sieber CC. Protein requirements in the elderly. Int J Vitam Nutr Res 2011;81(2–3):109–19.

18. Houston DK, Nicklas BJ, Ding J, et al. Dietary protein intake is associated with lean mass change in older, community-dwelling adults: the health, aging, and body composition (Health ABC) study. Am J Clin Nutr 2008;87(1):150–5.

19. Chan R, Leung J, Woo J, et al. Associations of dietary protein intake on subsequent decline in muscle mass and physical functions over four years in ambulant older Chinese people. J Nutr Health Aging 2014;18(2):171–7.

20. Kortebein P, Symons TB, Ferrando A, et al. Functional impact of 10 days of bed rest in healthy older adults. J Gerontol A Biol Sci Med Sci 2008;63(10):1076–81.

21. Bell KE, von Allmen MT, Devries MC, et al. Muscle disuse as a pivotal problem in sarcopenia-related muscle loss and dysfunction. J Frailty Aging 2016;5(1):33–41.

22. Visser M, Goodpaster BH, Kritchevsky SB, et al. Muscle mass, muscle strength, and muscle fat infiltration as predictors of incident mobility limitations in well-functioning older persons. J Gerontol A Biol Sci Med Sci 2005;60(3):324–33.

23. Lang T, Cauley JA, Tylavsky F, et al. Computed tomographic measurements of thigh muscle cross-sectional area and attenuation coefficient predict hip fracture: the health, aging, and body composition study. J Bone Miner Res 2010;25(3): 513–9.

24. Landi F, Liperoti R, Russo A, et al. Sarcopenia as a risk factor for falls in elderly individuals: results from the ilSIRENTE study. Clin Nutr 2012;31(5):652–8.

25. Yu R, Leung J, Woo J. Incremental predictive value of sarcopenia for incident fracture in an elderly Chinese cohort: results from the Osteoporotic Fractures in Men (MrOs) Study. J Am Med Dir Assoc 2014;15(8):551–8.

26. Chalhoub D, Cawthon PM, Ensrud KE, et al. Risk of nonspine fractures in older adults with sarcopenia, low bone mass, or both. J Am Geriatr Soc 2015;63(9): 1733–40.

27. Rantanen T, Guralnik JM, Foley D, et al. Midlife hand grip strength as a predictor of old age disability. JAMA 1999;281(6):558–60.

28. Al Snih S, Markides KS, Ottenbacher KJ, et al. Hand grip strength and incident ADL disability in elderly Mexican Americans over a seven-year period. Aging Clin Exp Res 2004;16(6):481–6.

29. Janssen I. Influence of sarcopenia on the development of physical disability: the Cardiovascular Health Study. J Am Geriatr Soc 2006;54(1):56–62.

30. Gale CR, Martyn CN, Cooper C, et al. Grip strength, body composition, and mortality. Int J Epidemiol 2007;36(1):228–35.

31. Prado CM, Wells JC, Smith SR, et al. Sarcopenic obesity: a critical appraisal of the current evidence. Clin Nutr 2012;31(5):583–601.

32. Auyeung TW, Lee JS, Leung J, et al. Adiposity to muscle ratio predicts incident physical limitation in a cohort of 3,153 older adults–an alternative measurement of sarcopenia and sarcopenic obesity. Age (Dordr) 2013;35(4):1377–85.

33. Atkins JL, Whincup PH, Morris RW, et al. Sarcopenic obesity and risk of cardio-vascular disease and mortality: a population-based cohort study of older men. J Am Geriatr Soc 2014;62(2):253–60.

34. Fried LP, Tangen CM, Walston J, et al. Frailty in older adults: evidence for a phenotype. J Gerontol A Biol Sci Med Sci 2001;56(3):M146–56.

35. Mitnitski AB, Mogilner AJ, Rockwood K. Accumulation of deficits as a proxy mea-sure of aging. ScientificWorldJournal 2001;1:323–36.

36. Evans WJ, Morley JE, Argiles J, et al. Cachexia: a new definition. Clin Nutr 2008; 27(6):793–9.

37. Yu R, Leung J, Woo J. Sarcopenia combined with FRAX probabilities improves fracture risk prediction in older Chinese men. J Am Med Dir Assoc 2014; 15(12):918–23.

38. Andrews NA. The muscle–bone connection. IBMS BoneKEy 2013;10 (Article no: 377).

39. Woo J, Leung J, Morley JE. Defining sarcopenia in terms of incident adverse out-comes. J Am Med Dir Assoc 2015;16(3):247–52.

40. Woo J, Leung J, Morley JE. Validating the SARC-F: a suitable community screening tool for sarcopenia? J Am Med Dir Assoc 2014;15(9):630–4.

41. Malmstrom TK, Miller DK, Simonsick EM, et al. SARC-F: a symptom score to pre-dict persons with sarcopenia at risk for poor functional outcomes. J Cachexia Sar-copenia Muscle 2016;7(1):28–36.

42. Landi F, Martone AM, Calvani R, et al. Sarcopenia risk screening tool: a new strat-egy for clinical practice. J Am Med Dir Assoc 2014;15(9):613–4.

43. Trabal J, Forga M, Leyes P, et al. Effects of free leucine supplementation and resistance training on muscle strength and functional status in older adults: a ran-domized controlled trial. Clin Interv Aging 2015;10:713–23.

44. Nelson ME, Rejeski WJ, Blair SN, et al. Physical activity and public health in older adults: recommendation from the American College of Sports Medicine and the American Heart Association. Med Sci Sports Exerc 2007;39(8):1435–45.

45. Williams MA, Haskell WL, Ades PA, et al. Resistance exercise in individuals with and without cardiovascular disease: 2007 update: a scientific statement from the American Heart Association Council on Clinical Cardiology and Council on Nutri-tion, Physical Activity, and Metabolism. Circulation 2007;116(5):572–84.

46. Cadore EL, Casas-Herrero A, Zambom-Ferraresi F, et al. Multicomponent exer-cises including muscle power training enhance muscle mass, power output, and functional outcomes in institutionalized frail nonagenarians. Age (Dordr) 2014;36(2):773–85.

47. Kraemer RR, Castracane VD. Novel insights regarding mechanisms for treatment of sarcopenia. Metabolism 2015;64(2):160–2.

48. Rolland Y, Onder G, Morley JE, et al. Current and future pharmacologic treatment of sarcopenia. Clin Geriatr Med 2011;27(3):423–47.

49. Parise G, Snijders T. Myostatin inhibition for treatment of sarcopenia. Lancet Dia-betes Endocrinol 2015;3(12):917–8.

50. Drescher C, Konishi M, Ebner N, et al. Loss of muscle mass: current develop-ments in cachexia and sarcopenia focused on biomarkers and treatment. Int J Cardiol 2016;202:766–72.

51. Studenski S. Clinical and biological markers of sarcopenia: where are we? J Frailty Aging 2012;1(3):1–2.

Anorexia of Aging
Assessment and Management

Francesco Landi, MD, PhD*, Anna Picca, PhD, Riccardo Calvani, PhD,
Emanuele Marzetti, MD, PhD

KEYWORDS

- Weight loss • Cachexia • Sarcopenia • Nutrition • Appetite • Food intake
- Multidimensional intervention • Geriatric syndrome

KEY POINTS

- Anorexia is common in advanced age and is associated with multiple adverse health outcomes, including reduced quality of life, morbidity, and mortality.
- Anorexia of aging results from the various contributions of alterations of peripheral and central regulatory systems, medications, comorbidities, and psychosocial factors.
- Eating habits and nutritional status should be routinely evaluated to identify older persons with appetite disturbances who are at risk of developing malnutrition.
- Multidimensional strategies, involving food manipulation, targeted nutritional supplementation, and psychosocial support, are effective at preventing and treating anorexia and its negative outcomes.

INTRODUCTION

Food intake undergoes substantial changes over the life course,[1] implying variations in body energy fuel reservoirs. Being essential for the execution of any activity, the preservation of overall bodily energy status is critical for successful aging. Indeed, a breach in the nutritional status makes older adults more vulnerable to internal and/or external stressors, which can severely affect overall health and quality of life.

Disclosure Statement: R. Calvani, F. Landi, and E. Marzetti are partners of the SPRINTT Consortium, which is partly funded by the European Federation of Pharmaceutical Industries and Associations (EFPIA). A. Picca declares no conflict of interest.
The study was partly supported by grants from the Innovative Medicines Initiative – Joint Undertaking (IMI-JU #115621), intramural research grants from the Catholic University of the Sacred Heart (D3.2 2013 and D3.2 2015), Fondazione Roma (NCDs Call for Proposals 2013), and the nonprofit research foundation "Centro Studi Achille e Linda Lorenzon."
Department of Geriatrics, Neurosciences and Orthopedics, Center for Geriatric Medicine (CEMI), Institute of Internal Medicine and Geriatrics, Catholic University of the Sacred Heart, L.go F. Vito 8, Rome 00168, Italy
* Corresponding author.
E-mail address: francesco.landi@unicatt.it

The term "anorexia of aging" has been coined to indicate the multifactorial decrease in appetite and/or food intake occurring in late life.[2] Because malnutrition represents the endpoint of the mismatch between dietary intake and energy demands, this disorder has been recognized as a specific geriatric syndrome that can lead to malnutrition if not appropriately diagnosed and treated.[3,4]

In addition to alterations of the nutritional status, other relevant clinical correlates of anorexia of aging include body wasting (ie, cachexia and sarcopenia), poor endurance, reduced physical performance, slow gait speed, and impaired mobility.[2,5] Selective nutritional deficits can impact the health status also in the absence of overt malnutrition. For instance, insufficient protein intake increases the risk of developing sarcopenia and is associated with morbidity and mortality.[6–9] In addition, anorexia has been shown to impact survival in older adults independent of age, gender, and multimorbidity.[10,11]

Although nutritional counseling should be considered at any stage as a key element to preserve good health, special efforts should be directed to increasing awareness of health care providers about nutritional disorders specific to the elderly. In addition, attention should be given to older people in acute and post-acute care settings, as they are at higher risk of incurring adverse health outcomes. As such, the adoption of nutritional evaluations as a routine component of geriatric assessment needs to be prioritized to facilitate therapeutic decision making.[12,13]

In this review, we provide a concise synopsis on the multiple causes and factors composing the biological substrate of anorexia of aging, as well as some of the risk factors associated with this condition with a special emphasis on the current available tools for its assessment and management.

ANOREXIA OF AGING: THE BIOLOGICAL SUBSTRATE

The complex pathophysiology of anorexia of aging resides in its multifactorial origin involving derangements of both peripheral and central regulatory systems.[14] Several factors, including age-related gradual decrease in smell and taste perception, hormonal changes in gut mediators (for example, cholecystokinin [CCK], glucagon-like peptide 1), and altered secretion pattern of ghrelin after nutrient intake, affect satiation and dietary behaviors.[2] All these factors modulate the function and activity of central regulatory systems both indirectly via activation of afferent vagal fibers and directly through releasing neurotransmitters into the blood.

In particular, alterations of the sense of taste and smell, occurring after the age of 50 to 60 years, contributes to reducing food palatability and impacts diet variety. On the other hand, the "hunger hormone" ghrelin released by the gastrointestinal mucosa is negatively modulated by circulating leptin and insulin, the levels of which may be altered in older adults.[15–18] Similar to ghrelin, modifications in the dynamics of CCK have also been observed in advanced age and associated with anorexia of aging.[15–18] Interestingly, age-related increases in CCK and peptide YY circulating levels have been shown to convey synergistic anorexigenic signals to the hypothalamus.[15–18]

Gastrointestinal muscular tone and motility both decrease during aging. As a consequence, older people may experience longer-lasting satiety due to delayed gastric emptying. Slower gastrointestinal transit also favors constipation and flatulence, further contributing to reducing food desire. In addition, diminished stomach digestive ability, enhanced and prolonged antral distension, and modifications of small intestine satiety signals in older individuals may further decrease appetite and food intake in old age.[15–18]

Finally, age-related chronic low-grade inflammation may alter the response of specific brain areas to peripheral stimuli via the action of circulating mediators, including interleukin (IL)-1, IL-6, and tumor necrosis factor-α, that are typically increased in older persons.[19] The reduction of food intake and body weight caused by inflammatory cytokine signaling seems to be mostly due to their effect on gastric emptying and clampdown of small intestinal motility.[19] In addition, these inflammatory mediators directly stimulate leptin expression and enhance circulating leptin levels,[19,20] and instigate the production of hypothalamic corticotropin-releasing factor, a mediator of the anorexigenic effect of leptin.[19,21]

All the previously mentioned factors are particularly relevant to the management of anorexia of aging, because their knowledge may allow for the development and implementation of novel preventive and therapeutic strategies.

RISK FACTORS

The development of anorexia of aging is influenced by comorbid conditions that directly or indirectly interfere with nutritional status. Functional impairment, social and environmental conditions, acute and chronic diseases, and their treatments represent only a few risk factors associated with age-related weight loss.[22] In particular, physical limitations, leading to mobility problems, induce functional impairments in activities of daily living (eg, inability to eating independently, difficulty in getting foods, inability to cook) that easily instigate reduced food intake and malnourishment.[5] In this context, also sensory impairment (hearing and vision) may affect the ability of older people to perform standard daily activities (eg, do grocery shopping, prepare, and consume food).

Other physical factors, such as poor dentition, poor-fitting prosthesis, or inflammatory states of the oral cavity, may limit the type and quantity of food intake. Problems with chewing and swallowing directly correlate with poor intake of nutrients like proteins, fibers, vitamins, and calcium, while favoring higher intake of fats and cholesterol.[22,23]

Several age-related common conditions/diseases alter appetite and produce malabsorption or increased energy expenditure. This is, for instance, the case of malabsorption syndromes, gastrointestinal diseases, acute and chronic infections, and hypermetabolism (eg, hyperthyroidism), representing major candidates for micronutrient deficiencies, loss of appetite, reduced food intake, and ultimately anorexia, in the face of increased energy requirements.[4,24,25]

Other chronic conditions like cancer and inflammatory diseases, such as rheumatoid arthritis, which are highly prevalent in late life, induce anorectic effects via proinflammatory signaling. Both anorexia and fat malabsorption, as well as fat-losing enteropathy are common in advanced heart failure.[24] In addition, chronic obstructive pulmonary disease causes anorexia as a consequence of oxygen deprivation and increased metabolism due to heightened activity of respiratory muscles.[24]

Alterations of nutritional status have been described as a consequence of several drug prescriptions, as well as over-the-counter medications that older people often take.[26] Medications like digoxin and antiblastic drugs can cause nausea, vomiting, and loss of appetite. Penicillamine, by inducing zinc decrease, can lead to loss of taste acuity, and high doses of antiacids containing aluminum or magnesium hydroxide deplete phosphate and potassium storage. Polypharmacy, which is highly common among older people, further increases the risk of drug-induced anorexia, due to high odds of drug-drug interactions and gastrointestinal problems.[26]

Another relevant condition often associated with loss of appetite is depression, one of the most common age-related psychological disorders.[14] Older people diagnosed with depression seem to suffer more severe appetite reduction and weight loss than younger counterparts. Depressed elderly, especially nursing home residents, have numerous symptoms and signs that can contribute to anorexia and weight loss, including weakness, stomach ache, nausea, and diarrhea.[14] Even more worrisome is that, in older persons with major depression, denial to eat may represent a suicidal gesture. In these individuals, indeed, eating refusal represents an ethically acceptable method to exit life. Finally, depression is associated with an increased cerebrospinal fluid concentration of corticotropin-releasing factor that acts as a potent anorectic agent.

Cognitive impairment is associated with loss of appetite and reduced food intake. As many as 50% of institutionalized elderly individuals with any kind of dementia show protein-energy malnutrition. The occurrence of anorexia in older adults with dementia is related mainly to difficulty with swallowing (dysphagia; "apraxia of swallowing") and behavioral disorders, such as wandering and resistance to care.[24,25] Although some elderly individuals with dementia increase their energy expenditure by continuing walking, unintentional and significant weight loss is mainly attributed to failure to eat regularly.

Several social factors also can put older persons at risk of malnutrition. Economic inequality represents a relevant factor. Indeed, older individuals with inadequate financial means often experience problems with obtaining good-quality foods, thereby affecting nutrient intake in terms of variety and macronutrient and micronutrient composition.[27] Social isolation is another major factor contributing to the development of anorexia of aging. Living alone per se is associated with decreased appetite and energy intake, and older individuals tend to ingest more food (up to 50%) and energy during a meal when eating in the company of others.[27] Poor education on adequate nutritional needs also can result in insufficient dietary intake with insufficient variety of food choices. Lack of knowledge on the possible detrimental effects of dietary restriction may in some cases lead an older person to assume a semistarvation regimen. Finally, among institutionalized older individuals, anorexia and subsequent unintentional weight loss can be the consequence of the monotony and repetitiousness of daily foods.[2] Failure by the institution to pay attention to personal food preferences and to stimulate a favorable environment to eat are important factors related to loss of appetite and reduced food intake among nursing home residents.

ASSESSMENT AND MANAGEMENT OF ANOREXIA OF AGING

Given the negative health outcomes associated with anorexia of aging, the evaluation of the nutritional status and the identification of risk factors for malnutrition always should be included as part of older patient assessment. To date, validated screening tools exist that are available to identify anorexia in older persons or at risk for it. Among these, the Simplified Nutritional Assessment Questionnaire (SNAQ) is a self-assessment nutritional screening tool that allows for identifying older people at risk of malnutrition or who are malnourished (**Table 1**).[28,29] The Functional Assessment of Anorexia and Cachexia Therapy shortened 12-question version (FAACT) questionnaire may be used to identify anorexia-related symptoms and grade their severity (**Table 2**).[30]

Multistep screening/assessment programs aimed at identifying and addressing risk factors for anorexia of aging are particularly useful for the management of anorexia (**Fig. 1**). The first step involves the identification of subjects at risk for developing the condition by using second- and third-generation geriatric assessment tools. The

Table 1
The Simplified Nutritional Assessment Questionnaire (SNAQ)

	A	B	C	D	E
My appetite is:	Very poor	Poor	Average	Good	Very good
When I eat:	I feel full after eating only a few mouthfuls	I feel full after eating about a third of a meal	I feel full after eating over half a meal	I feel full after eating most of the meal	I hardly ever feel full
Food tastes:	Very bad	Bad	Average	Good	Very good
Normally I eat:	Less than 1 meal a day	One meal a day	Two meals a day	Three meals a day	More than 3 meals a day

This tool is based on the following scoring system: A = 1; B = 2; C = 3; D = 4; E = 5. SNAQ scores ≤14 indicate significant risk of at least 5% weight loss within 6 months.
From Wilson MM, Thomas DR, Rubenstein LZ, et al. Appetite assessment: simple appetite questionnaire predicts weight loss in community-dwelling adults and nursing home residents. Am J Clin Nutr 2005;82(5):1074–81; with permission.

Minimum Data Set-Inter Resident Assessment Suite represents a powerful suite of comprehensive geriatric assessment instruments that cover a wide spectrum of clinical, psychological, socioeconomic, and environmental factors across different health care settings.[12] Independent of the assessment tool adopted, once an anorectic condition is identified, adjustments in feeding patterns may be sufficient in milder cases, whereas a thorough dietary revision is required in more advanced cases. After an intervention has been implemented, follow-up assessments should be carried out to evaluate the efficacy of the treatment plan and program future actions (see **Fig. 1**).[31]

Table 2
Functional assessment of anorexia and cachexia therapy shortened 12-question version (FAACT) questionnaire

	0	1	2	3	4
The amount I eat is sufficient to meet my needs					
I have a good appetite					
I am worried about my weight					
Most food tastes unpleasant to me					
I am concerned about how thin I look					
My interest in food drops as soon as I try to eat					
I have difficulty eating rich or "heavy" foods					
My family or friends are pressuring me to eat					
I have been vomiting					
When I eat, I seem to get full quickly					
I have pain in my stomach area					
My general health is improving					

This tool is based on the following scoring system: 0 = Not at all; 1 = A little bit; 2 = Somewhat; 3 = Quite a bit; 4 = Very much. A score of 24 indicates the presence of anorexia.
From Davis MP, Yavuzsen T, Kirkova J, et al. Validation of a simplified anorexia questionnaire. J Pain Symptom Manage 2009;38(5):691–7; with permission.

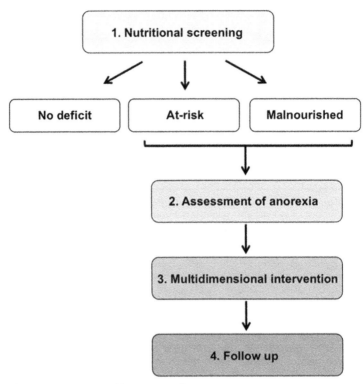

Fig. 1. Multistep anorexia/nutrition care pathway.

TREATMENT OPTIONS FOR ANOREXIA OF AGING

The optimal management of older persons with anorexia requires a comprehensive intervention and the preliminary elimination of all potentially reversible contributing factors. Food manipulation, correction of environmental and pharmacologic risk factors, and treatment of comorbidities are among the actions to be pursued.[24,32,33] In particular, food manipulation implies the optimization of food texture and palatability, flavor enhancement, dietary variety, and feeding assistance as needed, whereas environmental interventions rely on the promotion of conviviality, especially in institutionalized elderly. Given the impact several pharmacologic therapies have in decreasing appetite and favoring weight loss, a thorough evaluation of prescription and over-the-counter medications is crucial. Cardiovascular (eg, digoxin, amiodarone, and spironolactone), psychotropic (eg, phenothiazines, lithium, amitriptyline, fluoxetine, and other selective serotonin reuptake inhibitors), and antirheumatic drugs (nonsteroidal anti-inflammatory agents) are the most commonly prescribed medications that may interfere with appetite.[2]

Comorbidities that can contribute to weight loss need to be adequately addressed. This is the case in swallowing disorders (eg, dry mouth, tooth loss, mouth lesions), dyspepsia (eg, gastritis and ulcer), malabsorption syndromes (eg, bacterial overgrowth, gluten enteropathy, pancreatic insufficiency), neurologic disorders (eg, stroke), endocrine disorders (eg, hyperparathyroidism), psychiatric disorders (eg, depression, delirium), respiratory diseases (eg, chronic obstructive pulmonary disease), and cardiovascular diseases (eg, congestive heart failure).[2]

No therapeutic agents are to date available for treating anorexia of aging. Few studies have shown positive effects of nutritional supplementation in malnourished older adults, but the heterogeneity of intervention protocol hinders their applicability in clinical practice. The only robust evidence in support of nutritional supplementation in older adults regards protein supplementation. In particular, a daily intake of 1.0 to 1.2 g of protein per kilogram of body weight has been proposed to prevent the loss of muscle mass and strength.[34]

Several drugs have been tested for the stimulation of appetite in older adults with anorexia, but none of them has shown successful outcomes that may support their implementation in clinical practice.[24,32,33] For instance, corticosteroids induce gains in body weight, primarily via increasing fluid retention. Growth hormone administration also favors weight gain in malnourished older individuals, but without functional improvements. The administration of anabolic steroids (eg, testosterone and oxandrolone) has shown some beneficial effects, but side effects (eg, cardiovascular events and liver dysfunction) offset benefits.[2] The same limitations affect metoclopramide that, although reducing early satiety in some patients, is associated with extrapyramidal signs and symptoms with long-term use. Other appetite-stimulating drugs (eg, megestrol, moclobemide, tetrahydrocannabinol, cyproheptadine, CCK antagonists) have been associated with relevant side effects, such as delirium and abdominal symptoms.[2]

SUMMARY

The management of anorexia of aging is to date a challenge for geriatricians considering its impact on quality of life, morbidity, and mortality. Second-generation and third-generation geriatric assessment tools are effective at identifying older persons at higher risk for anorexia and malnourishment. Such instruments also allow discovering and possibly eliminating reversible factors that underlie anorexia, thereby preventing its progression toward malnutrition. In the absence of effective antianorectic drugs, multidimensional interventions within personalized care plans currently represent the only available option to ensure the provision of adequate amounts of food, limit weight loss, and prevent adverse health outcomes in older adults.

REFERENCES

1. Briefel RR, McDowell MA, Alaimo K, et al. Total energy intake of the US population: the third National Health and Nutrition Examination Survey, 1988-1991. Am J Clin Nutr 1995;62(5 Suppl):1072S–80S.

2. Landi F, Calvani R, Tosato M, et al. Anorexia of aging: risk factors, consequences, and potential treatments. Nutrients 2016;8(2):69.

3. Donini LM, Savina C, Piredda M, et al. Senile anorexia in acute-ward and rehabilitation settings. J Nutr Health Aging 2008;12(8):511–7.

4. MacIntosh C, Morley JE, Chapman IM. The anorexia of aging. Nutrition 2000; 16(10):983–95.

5. Landi F, Russo A, Liperoti R, et al. Anorexia, physical function, and incident disability among the frail elderly population: results from the ilSIRENTE study. J Am Med Dir Assoc 2010;11(4):268–74.

6. Landi F, Laviano A, Cruz-Jentoft AJ. The anorexia of aging: is it a geriatric syndrome? J Am Med Dir Assoc 2010;11(3):153–6.

7. Muscaritoli M, Anker SD, Argilés J, et al. Consensus definition of sarcopenia, cachexia and pre-cachexia: joint document elaborated by special interest groups

(SIG) "cachexia-anorexia in chronic wasting diseases" and "nutrition in geriatrics." Clin Nutr 2010;29(2):154–9.

8. Martone AM, Onder G, Vetrano DL, et al. Anorexia of aging: a modifiable risk factor for frailty. Nutrients 2013;5(10):4126–33.

9. Landi F, Liperoti R, Russo A, et al. Association of anorexia with sarcopenia in a community-dwelling elderly population: results from the ilSIRENTE study. Eur J Nutr 2013;52(3):1261–8.

10. Landi F, Liperoti R, Lattanzio F, et al. Effects of anorexia on mortality among older adults receiving home care: an observation study. J Nutr Health Aging 2012; 16(1):79–83.

11. Incalzi RA, Gemma A, Capparella O, et al. Energy intake and in-hospital starvation. A clinically relevant relationship. Arch Intern Med 1996;156(4):425–9.

12. Bernabei R, Landi F, Onder G, et al. Second and third generation assessment instruments: the birth of standardization in geriatric care. J Gerontol A Biol Sci Med Sci 2008;63(3):308–13.

13. Sloane PD, Ivey J, Helton M, et al. Nutritional issues in long-term care. J Am Med Dir Assoc 2008;9(7):476–85.

14. Wysokiński A, Sobów T, Kłoszewska I, et al. Mechanisms of the anorexia of aging—a review. Age (Dordr) 2015;37(4):9821.

15. Di Francesco V, Fantin F, Omizzolo F, et al. The anorexia of aging. Dig Dis 2007; 25(2):129–37.

16. Chapman IM. The anorexia of aging. Clin Geriatr Med 2007;23(4):735–56.

17. Chapman IM. Endocrinology of anorexia of ageing. Best Pract Res Clin Endocrinol Metab 2004;18(3):437–52.

18. Chapman IM, MacIntosh CG, Morley JE, et al. The anorexia of ageing. Biogerontology 2002;3(1–2):67–71.

19. Yeh SS, Blackwood K, Schuster MW. The cytokine basis of cachexia and its treatment: are they ready for prime time? J Am Med Dir Assoc 2008;9(4):219–36.

20. Laviano A, Meguid MM, Inui A, et al. Therapy insight: cancer anorexia-cachexia syndrome—when all you can eat is yourself. Nat Clin Pract Oncol 2005;2(3): 158–65.

21. Morley JE, Thomas DR. Anorexia and aging: pathophysiology. Nutrition 1999; 15(6):499–503.

22. Landi F, Lattanzio F, Dell'Aquila G, et al. Prevalence and potentially reversible factors associated with anorexia among older nursing home residents: results from the ULISSE project. J Am Med Dir Assoc 2013;14(2):119–24.

23. Mir F, Zafar F, Morley JE. Anorexia of aging: can we decrease protein energy undernutrition in the nursing home? J Am Med Dir Assoc 2013;14(2):77–9.

24. Morley JE. Pathophysiology of the anorexia of aging. Curr Opin Clin Nutr Metab Care 2013;16(1):27–32.

25. Morley JE. Anorexia of aging: physiologic and pathologic. Am J Clin Nutr 1997; 66(4):760–73.

26. Onder G, Landi F, Fusco D, et al. Recommendations to prescribe in complex older adults: results of the CRIteria to assess appropriate medication use among elderly complex patients (CRIME) project. Drugs Aging 2014;31(1):33–45.

27. de Castro JM. Age-related changes in spontaneous food intake and hunger in humans. Appetite 1993;21(3):255.

28. Wilson MM, Thomas DR, Rubenstein LZ, et al. Appetite assessment: simple appetite questionnaire predicts weight loss in community-dwelling adults and nursing home residents. Am J Clin Nutr 2005;82(5):1074–81.

29. Wilson MM, Thomas DR, Rubenstein LZ, et al. Appetite assessment: simple appetite questionnaire predicts weight loss in community-dwelling adults and nursing home residents. Am J Clin Nutr 2005;82(5):1074–81.

30. Davis MP, Yavuzsen T, Kirkova J, et al. Validation of a simplified anorexia questionnaire. J Pain Symptom Manage 2009;38(5):691–7.

31. Correia MI, Hegazi RA, Higashiguchi T, et al. Evidence-based recommendations for addressing malnutrition in health care: an updated strategy from the feedM.E. Global Study Group. J Am Med Dir Assoc 2014;15(8):544–50.

32. Morley JE. Anorexia of aging: a true geriatric syndrome. J Nutr Health Aging 2012;16(5):422–5.

33. Luca A, Luca M, Calandra C. Eating disorders in late-life. Aging Dis 2014;6(1):48–55.

34. Bauer J, Biolo G, Cederholm T, et al. Evidence-based recommendations for optimal dietary protein intake in older people: a position paper from the PROT-AGE Study Group. J Am Med Dir Assoc 2013;14(8):542–59.

Mild Cognitive Impairment

Angela M. Sanford, MD

KEYWORDS

- Mild cognitive impairment • MCI • Early dementia • Cognitive decline
- Memory impairment

KEY POINTS

- Mild cognitive impairment (MCI) occurs along a continuum with normal cognition at one end of the continuum and dementia at the other.
- Guidelines for universal screening have not been established, but would likely facilitate earlier diagnosis and treatment.
- MCI is not synonymous with Alzheimer disease and does not always progress to dementia.
- There are no approved pharmacologic treatments for MCI, but progression may be slowed or stopped with attention to treating reversible causes and making lifestyle changes.

INTRODUCTION

Mild cognitive impairment (MCI), first fully characterized by Petersen and associates in 1997,[1] generally refers to impairment in cognition above that which is seen with normal age-related cognitive decline, but not severe enough to cause significantly impaired daily function (**Fig. 1**). Clinically, the term "age-related cognitive decline" is synonymous with changes in memory and cognition that are characteristically seen with advancing age or "normal aging." Although there are 6 main cognitive domains that could potentially be affected (learning and memory, social functioning, language, visuospatial function, complex attention, or executive functioning),[2,3] the term "mild cognitive impairment" generally refers to a decline in the ability to learn new information or recall stored information. Keeping in mind these main cognitive domains, MCI can be further classified as "amnestic" versus "nonamnestic." Amnestic MCI refers to impairment purely in one's ability to recall stored information, whereas nonamnestic MCI refers to impairment in 1 or more of the other cognitive domains, while memory remains relatively intact.[4] Nonamnestic cognitive decline is comparatively less common and often more difficult to diagnose than the amnestic form of MCI.

The author has no financial disclosures, outside funding sources, or conflicts of interest.
Department of Internal Medicine-Geriatrics, Saint Louis University School of Medicine, 1402 South Grand Boulevard, Suite M238, St Louis, MO 63104, USA
E-mail address: lipkaa@slu.edu

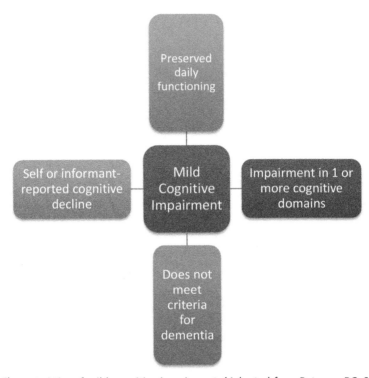

Fig. 1. Characteristics of mild cognitive impairment. (*Adapted from* Petersen RC, Smith GE, Waring SC, et al. Aging, memory and mild cognitive impairment. Int Psychogeriatr 1997;9 Suppl 1:65–9; with permission.)

Although not defined by earlier editions, the *Diagnostic and Statistical Manual of Mental Disorders 5th Edition* (DSM-V) classifies MCI as a "mild neurocognitive disorder," and specifies that there must be both a subjective and objective decline from previous level of functioning in 1 or more of the 6 cognitive domains, not substantially interfering with instrumental activities of daily living, and not occurring in the context of delirium or other psychological disorders.[3] Remarkably, none of the common definitions of MCI list advanced age as a criterion, although most of the research conducted in this area occurs in the geriatric population.[5] To further build on these definitions, MCI should be recognized as part of a spectrum, with normal cognition on 1 end of the spectrum and dementia on the other end. Most people undergo some degree of cognitive decline as they age, but MCI exceeds this "age-related" decline in cognition, yet does not meet the criteria for dementia. Not all cases of MCI are precursors to dementia and not all are progressive. Fortunately, many cases revert back into the range of normal cognition. It is not always possible to predict the course of MCI in individuals, but a main goal for clinicians should be screening and early diagnosis so that causative factors can be identified and treated, ideally, preventing or postponing potential progression to dementia.

EPIDEMIOLOGY

The prevalence of MCI in those greater than 65 years of age is thought to be around 3% to 22%,[6–8] depending on the demographics of the population studied. The true prevalence can be difficult to ascertain from studies, because "cutoff" scores for determining MCI are not yet standardized and definitions among studies may vary.[9] There are several risk factors that increase the risk for developing MCI, with age being the strongest. Other well-established risk factors include male sex,[6,10] presence of the apolipoprotein E allele,[11] family history of cognitive impairment, and the presence of vascular risk factors such as hypertension, hyperlipidemia, coronary artery disease, and stroke.[12] One study focusing on multimorbidity and development of MCI found that those participants with 4 or more chronic conditions, particularly 2 of the following—hypertension, hyperlipidemia, coronary artery disease, and osteoarthritis—had the highest risk of MCI.[13] Other chronic medical conditions, such as chronic obstructive pulmonary disease,[14] depression,[15] and diabetes mellitus,[16] are also known risk factors. Lifestyle plays a role as well, with those who are cognitively and/or physically sedentary at greater risk for developing MCI.[17,18]

Interestingly, studies have found quite high conversion rates, with 30% to 50% of those originally diagnosed with MCI reverting back to "normal" cognition at subsequent follow-up.[16,19–21] Some factors found to be associated with a greater likelihood of return to normal cognition include single domain impairment,[19,20] presence of depression,[22] use of anticholinergic medications,[22] absence of the apolipoprotein E ε4 allele,[16] greater hippocampal volume on neuroimaging,[23] and higher scores on cognitive testing.[16] Despite the high reversion rate, however, there is a 5% to 10% annual rate of progression to dementia in those with MCI, which is much higher than the 1% to 2% incidence per year among the general population.[24,25] This dichotomy between the annual reversion rate to normal cognition and the conversion rate to dementia indicates that there are modifiable factors that may be contributing to cognitive decline and makes the case for the necessity of early screening and diagnosis.

PATHOPHYSIOLOGY

In the past, MCI was thought simply to be "precursor" to or an "asymptomatic" phase of Alzheimer disease.[26] Although this can be true, in many cases, MCI does not further progress into dementia and there are many medical disorders known to have a positive association with MCI. These include Parkinson Disease, traumatic brain injury, cerebrovascular accident, Huntington disease, and human immunodeficiency virus.[2] Typically, with these diseases, the disease manifests first followed by cognitive impairment later in the disease course. In other instances, the cognitive impairment or behavioral symptoms manifest early in the disease course. This is typically seen with disorders primarily affecting cognition, such as Alzheimer disease, vascular dementia, Lewy body disease, prion disease, and frontotemporal dementia. In these disorders, there is often a prodromal stage representing MCI, which can often go undiagnosed. Unfortunately, the majority of these cases are progressive and ultimately result in dementia. In general, amnestic MCI, when it progresses to dementia, tends to develop into Alzheimer or vascular dementia, whereas nonamnestic MCI more commonly evolves into frontotemporal dementia or Lewy body disease.[27]

REVERSIBLE CAUSES

There are numerous treatable factors, when present, that can contribute to or even cause MCI (**Fig. 2**). These are often overlooked and underestimated, which is unfortunate, because some are easily fixable and will improve cognition greatly. One extremely influential factor impacting day-to-day cognition is polypharmacy. Many

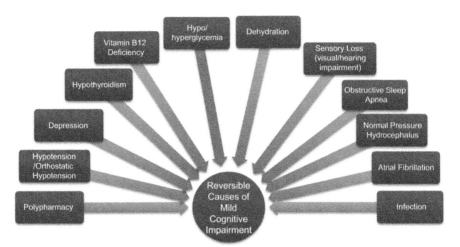

Fig. 2. Reversible causes of mild cognitive impairment.

common classes of medications can have subtle effects on memory, including opioids, muscle relaxants, anxiolytics, antiepileptics, and anticholinergic medications, which encompass antihistamine medications, antidepressants, antipsychotics, and urinary incontinence medications.[28,29] Antihypertensive medications may lead to relative hypotension and/or orthostatic hypotension, both of which can decrease cerebral blood flow and can make it difficult to think clearly.[30] One study found that cognitive scores were the highest around blood pressure levels of 135 mm Hg systolic, but decreased with lower blood pressures.[31] Each medication potentially has its own side effects and these side effects may be enhanced or compounded by drug–drug interactions between various medications.

Another frequently overlooked and common contributor to MCI is depression. Depression is a great conundrum and can cause impaired physical and cognitive functioning, leading the clinician down various diagnostic paths for answers. Cognition tends to clear once depression is addressed and treated adequately. Studies have also shown that depression can accelerate the conversion of MCI to dementia.[32,33] Metabolic deficiencies such as hypothyroidism,[34] hypoglycemia and hyperglycemia,[35] dehydration, and vitamin B_{12} deficiency[36] should all be assessed for and can be readily correctable, improving cognition. Atrial fibrillation may cause small, undetectable embolic events, mimicking small strokes or transient ischemic attacks, leading to MCI and ultimately vascular dementia.[37] Stroke risk in atrial fibrillation can be augmented with proper anticoagulation in those who are candidates. Obstructive sleep apnea is another correctable medical illness that can cause daytime fatigue and cognitive impairment when untreated.[38] Even sensory deficits such as visual and hearing loss may result in cognitive impairment and poor performance on cognitive testing.[39] The majority of cases can be improved with new glasses, cataract surgery, or hearing aids. Normal pressure hydrocephalus, which is an accumulation of cerebrospinal fluid (CSF) in the brain's ventricular system that causes ventricular enlargement and ultimately brain damage, can affect the ability to recall information. Hallmark symptoms include the triad of impaired cognition, gait ataxia, and urinary incontinence. Often, the detrimental cognitive effects can be reversible if detected and treated early in the disease course.[40]

SCREENING AND DIAGNOSIS

It can be quite difficult to diagnose MCI from the cognitive decline or "forgetfulness" that is consistent with normal aging. Typically, the diagnosis is made after a patient or accompanying informant lodge a subjective complaint of the patient forgetting important events, conversations, dates, or phone numbers. The clinician will often then perform an objective test and the diagnosis is established. There is controversy over whether this case-finding approach is the most appropriate way to diagnose MCI or whether universal screening should occur and, perhaps, diagnoses made in earlier stages. The International Association of Gerontology and Geriatrics released a consensus paper in 2015 that recommended that all persons 70 years and older have annual subjective or objective cognitive testing with their health care provider.[41] Although many clinicians and researchers are advocating for universal screening, guidelines have not been yet well-established and isolated case-finding continues to occur. It is also important to conduct a thorough workup for reversible causes, including screening for depression and obstructive sleep apnea, review of medications for those potentially affecting cognition, and laboratory assessment for vitamin B_{12} deficiency and hypothyroidism.

Cognitive impairment at all levels is severely underdiagnosed and undertreated by primary care physicians in community settings. In fact, it has been shown that, in patients with some degree of cognitive decline, it is not recognized and/or not documented by their primary care physicians in more than one-half of these patients.[42] That being said, it is quite time consuming to delve into a patient's history of cognitive decline, which encompasses cognition at previous baseline, changes that have occurred along the way, and current functioning level. Often, collateral information from family members is needed to establish a timeline so that an accurate diagnosis can be made. Not to mention, the time that is required to administer evidenced-based assessments and, once a diagnosis is established, the time needed to work the patient up for possible reversible causes. Primary care physicians are undertrained and frequently lack the time and support staff to accurately detect and address MCI. On some levels, Medicare recognizes these time and financial constraints and has introduced the Medicare Annual Wellness Visit, with the main goal of focusing on preventative services. This annual visit does reimburse primary care physicians for cognitive screening and would be an ideal visit to initiate universal cognitive screening.

Screening Instruments

Ideally, a formal diagnosis of MCI should be made after the administration of a standardized cognitive assessment. There are numerous screening tools that can be used, but we will focus here on the Saint Louis University Mental Status Examination (SLUMS), Rapid Cognitive Screen, and the Montreal Cognitive Assessment. The SLUMS is a 30-point questionnaire that takes less than 10 minutes to administer and is highly validated for diagnosing both MCI and dementia (**Fig. 3**). In comparison with the formerly commonly used Mini Mental Status Examination, the SLUMS has been found to be more sensitive in the detection of MCI and scoring is also adjusted for educational level,[43] which is an important component, because those with limited education cannot be expected to perform as well on cognitive tests as their more educated counterparts. Additionally, the SLUMs has been translated into 24 languages and is not copyrighted, unlike the Mini Mental Status Examination; thus, there is no charge for using it. The Rapid Cognitive Screen is a 10-point questionnaire developed from the SLUMs that takes less than 5 minutes to administer, making it convenient to administer in a busy clinical setting. It is likely not quite as sensitive as the SLUMS in the detection of MCI, but can be used when there are time constraints.[44]

VAMC
SLUMS Examination

Questions about this assessment tool? E-mail aging@slu.edu.

Name _____ Age _____
Is patient alert? _____ Level of education _____

Department of
Veterans Affairs

_/1 ❶ 1. What day of the week is it?
_/1 ❶ 2. What is the year?
_/1 ❶ 3. What state are we in?
     4. Please remember these five objects. I will ask you what they are later.
         Apple   Pen   Tie   House   Car
     5. You have $100 and you go to the store and buy a dozen apples for $3 and a tricycle for $20.
      ❶   How much did you spend?
_/3 ❷   How much do you have left?
     6. Please name as many animals as you can in one minute.
_/3   ❶ 0-4 animals ❶ 5-9 animals ❷ 10-14 animals ❸ 15+ animals
_/5 7. What were the five objects I asked you to remember? 1 point for each one correct.
     8. I am going to give you a series of numbers and I would like you to give them to me backwards.
        For example, if I say 42, you would say 24.
_/2   ❶ 87   ❶ 649   ❶ 8537
     9. This is a clock face. Please put in the hour markers and the time at
        ten minutes to eleven o'clock.
     ❷ Hour markers okay
_/4 ❷ Time correct
_/2 ❶ 10. Please place an X in the triangle.

     ❶   Which of the above figures is largest?

     11. I am going to tell you a story. Please listen carefully because afterwards, I'm going to ask you
         some questions about it.
         Jill was a very successful stockbroker. She made a lot of money on the stock market. She then met
         Jack, a devastatingly handsome man. She married him and had three children. They lived in Chicago.
         She then stopped work and stayed at home to bring up her children. When they were teenagers, she
         went back to work. She and Jack lived happily ever after.
     ❷ What was the female's name?   ❷ What work did she do?
_/8 ❷ When did she go back to work?   ❷ What state did she live in?

_____   TOTAL SCORE

Department of
Veterans Affairs

SAINT LOUIS
UNIVERSITY

SCORING		
HIGH SCHOOL EDUCATION		**LESS THAN HIGH SCHOOL EDUCATION**
27-30	Normal	25-30
21-26	MNCD[a]	20-24
1-20	Dementia	1-19

Fig. 3. Saint Louis University mental status examination. [a] Mild Neurocognitive Disorder. (*From* Tariq SH, Tumosa N, Chibnall JT, et al. Comparison of the Saint Louis University mental status examination and the mini-mental state examination for detecting dementia and mild neurocognitive disorder—a pilot study. Am J Geriatr Psychiatry 2006;14:900–10; with permission.)

The Montreal Cognitive Assessment is similar to the SLUMS in that it is a 30-point questionnaire that takes approximately 10 minutes to administer and is available in numerous languages. It was actually originally validated for the purpose of detecting MCI and is also more sensitive (although less specific) than the Mini Mental Status Examination in capturing MCI.[45]

The DSM-V does not specify a particular screening test that should be used for diagnosis, but in general, scores need to fall 1 to 2 standard deviations below age- and education-adjusted normative means on cognitive testing for a diagnosis of MCI to be considered. More in-depth neuropsychological testing (as opposed to bedside clinical assessment) is ideal in many cases, and can delineate specifics on which cognitive domains are affected and can also quantify level of deficit, but is not always necessary. Neuropsychological testing can additionally aid in distinguishing memory impairment from normal aging and is particularly useful in cases where the deficits are quite subtle.

Imaging Studies and Biomarkers

After a diagnosis of MCI is made, it is essential to try to establish the etiology of the cognitive decline and evaluate the possibility of any reversible causes that may be contributing and which may be correctable. A standard workup includes MRI or computerized tomography, which can be useful in evaluating overall brain structure and ruling out conditions such as brain tumors, normal pressure hydrocephalus, vascular malformation, and strokes. They may also reveal white matter hyperintensities or ischemic small vessel changes, which can be valuable in distinguishing cognitive impairment from vascular dementia versus that from other causes. When vascular changes are noted, ensuring optimal control of risk factors such as hypertension, hyperlipidemia, tobacco use, diabetes mellitus, and atrial fibrillation is important to slow or prevent cognitive decline.

Another helpful, but not readily available imaging study that evaluates brain function, rather than structure is the PET scan with F-fluorodeoxyglucose. This particular scan, still done primarily for research purposes, involves administering a radioactive tracer, which is a marker of glucose metabolism and binds to highly active areas in the brain that are readily using glucose. Patients with areas of glucose hypometabolism in their temporal or parietal lobes, which can be synonymous with neurodegeneration, may be at higher risk of progression from MCI to dementia.[46] Additionally, FDG-PET is more sensitive than simple MRI imaging in the diagnosis of "early" dementia consistent with MCI.[47] Similarly, single-photon emission computed tomography (SPECT) uses a radioactive tracer to measure regional cerebral blood flow. This is an indirect measurement of brain activity, because cerebral perfusion is increased in very metabolically active areas and decreased in areas of neurodegeneration and decreased synaptic activity. FDG-PET imaging is more sensitive than SPECT in detecting MCI, but SPECT is more cost effective and more readily available than FDG-PET.[48]

Biomarkers are measurable indicators of specific pathologic disease processes and are used primarily in clinical trials or research settings, because there is lack of standardization in technique and uncertainty regarding optimal cutoff points for diagnosis. The most commonly used biomarkers were initially developed for early detection of Alzheimer disease and thus are specific for the core Alzheimer disease pathology of amyloid-rich plaque deposition and neurodegeneration. CSF measurements of amyloid proteins are available and represent 1 type of biomarker. As amyloid-rich plaques are deposited in the brain, lower levels are detected in the CSF and these low CSF levels have been show to be correlated positively with the progression of MCI to dementia.[49] Additionally, tau protein plays a key role in the pathology of Alzheimer disease and is the main constituent of the characteristic neurofibrillary tangles that disrupt neuronal function. CSF levels of tau protein are increased in patients with Alzheimer disease and have also been shown to be positive predictors in the conversion of MCI to dementia.[50]

Specific radioactive tracers that bind to beta-amyloid plaques in the brain have also been developed and are used in conjunction with PET imaging. These beta-amyloid plaques are typically seen in patients with Alzheimer disease, but their presence is not specific to Alzheimer disease, because amyloid deposits are found in other disease processes and also in healthy elderly patients without cognitive changes. The Alzheimer's Association has established criteria for appropriate usage of amyloid PET imaging in the following groups: patients with persistent or progressive unexplained MCI, patients with possible Alzheimer disease with an atypical clinical presentation, or patients with progressive dementia and early age of onset.[51] Amyloid PET imaging should not be used in asymptomatic individuals, those with a typical progressive dementia, for use in determining severity of cognitive impairment, or in patients with known apolipoprotein E allele.[51]

The risk of progression of dementia can also be correlated with hippocampal volume, which is determined on imaging studies and is an indicator of neurodegeneration. Those with MCI who have a hippocampal volume at or below the 25th percentile have a 2 to 3 time higher risk of progression of dementia in comparison to those with hippocampal measurements at or above the 75th percentile.[52] The quantification of hippocampal volume on imaging studies is not readily available at all imaging centers or institutions, because only highly trained neuroradiologists are able to read these studies accurately.

At the present time, MCI is essentially a clinical diagnosis and cannot be made based on laboratory tests or imaging alone. Specialized testing and imaging can augment clinical assessment and determine differential diagnoses between the various types of dementia,[53] which may allow for better prognostication and opportunity for patient and family education. Changes in the anatomy and physiology of the brain are likely present years before the emergence of clinically detectable symptoms, but biomarkers and specialized imaging studies are not done as routine screening owing to high costs and lack of standardized techniques and measures. Consequently, one must rely primarily on clinical acumen, unfortunately, usually after the disease process is well-established. Serial clinical assessments are often necessary to document decline and can be helpful in predicting rate of decline in individual cases as well.

Why Is Early Diagnosis Important?

Early screening and diagnosis of MCI is important for many reasons, the first being that early detection of cognitive decline can put interventions in place before further damage occurs and may postpone or even prevent progression to dementia. It also allows for ample time for the patient and family to plan ahead for the unknown and allows the patient to engage in shared decision making. The patient can be encouraged to sign paperwork to appoint a durable power of attorney for both health care and financial matters in the event he or she becomes unable to make decisions. It can also give the patient and family time to establish a sound plan for "aging in place" and the patient can help to lay down the framework so that his or her wishes and desires are upheld. Importantly, early diagnosis can encourage family education and patient–family communication, and provide both justification and validation for the patient's abilities and behaviors. Potentially risky situations, such as driving, gun safety, susceptibility to financial scams, and so on, can be addressed before they occur and avoidance plans established. Finally, early diagnosis can allow the patient to participate in research studies and community support groups if desired.

TREATMENT

First and foremost, it cannot be stressed enough that evaluating for and treating the reversible causes of MCI will yield the most positive results and have the most beneficial effects on cognition. Focusing on treating depression, hypothyroidism, obstructive sleep apnea, hypotension, and polypharmacy could potentially lead to reversion of MCI back to normal cognition. Additionally, optimizing risk factors such as hypertension, hyperlipidemia, atrial fibrillation, tobacco use, and diabetes mellitus is essential and may slow down any further ischemic damage, halting the progression of MCI.[54] MCI is not always "curable" and treatments may be deemed successful if they slow the progression of the disease rather than reverse the cognitive changes.

Currently, there are no pharmacologic treatments approved by the Food and Drug Administration (FDA) for treatment of MCI, so the focus for treatment has shifted to factors such as diet, exercise, and cognitive stimulation. Multiple trials have been conducted looking at the effects of cholinesterase inhibitors (ie, donepezil, rivastigmine, galantamine) on MCI and progression to dementia, because this class of medication is Federal Drug Administration approved for the treatment of mild to moderate Alzheimer dementia. Unfortunately, their effects in MCI were null and they have not been found to delay the onset of dementia.[55,56] Accepting the risk of side effects such as orthostatic hypotension, falls, diarrhea, nausea, fatigue, and bradycardia with these medications is not warranted if no benefit has been seen. Additionally disappointing are the studies conducted with various antioxidants, vitamins, and supplements, such as vitamin E,[57] vitamin C,[58] vitamin B_{12},[59] ginko biloba,[60] and multivitamins.[61] There seems to be no benefit on cognition with supplementation unless there is a clear vitamin deficiency. Cognition in those found to have low serum levels of vitamin B_{12} does improve with vitamin B_{12} supplementation.[62] The antioxidant vitamins likely only target 1 small pathway of the numerous pathways involved in the pathologic changes causing dementia and thus do not influence the overall disease course.

There are several lifestyle modifications that have shown promising results in slowing the progression of MCI. Those that consume the "Mediterranean diet," which is a diet rich in plant-based foods such as legumes, whole grains, nuts, red wine, fish, and monounsaturated fats have a lower incidence of cognitive impairment[63] and studies have shown that consistently following this diet can actually slow the decline in MCI.[64] Physical exercise is highly protective against cognitive decline with a metaanalysis of 15 cohort studies revealing a 38% risk reduction of cognitive decline in participants who were physically active in comparison with their sedentary counterparts.[65] The exact mechanisms behind this risk reduction are unknown, but it is thought that exercise stimulates nutrient and oxygen-rich blood flow to the brain, protects against cardiovascular/cerebrovascular disease, reduces stress and cortisol levels, and also stimulates the release of neurotrophins, promoting optimal neuronal health.[66]

Not only is physical activity neuroprotective, but engaging in meaningful mental stimulation and intellectual activity also protects against the development of MCI and even improves cognition.[67] Examples of meaningful activities include doing crossword puzzles, word seek-and-find puzzles, or jigsaw puzzles, playing card games, playing an instrument, or socializing with others. Cognitive stimulation therapy is an evidence-based group intervention developed in the United Kingdom to stimulate and engage those with dementia, while providing socialization. It has been shown to improve cognition and quality of life in participants.[68] Modules have yet to be developed for patients with MCI and it is unknown if the responses would be similar for those with less impaired cognition, but in theory, cognitive stimulation therapy would likely be beneficial for those with MCI, because it encourages social engagement, learning, and recall. For better or worse, most of the available "treatments" for MCI rely heavily on patient motivation and participation. Aside from the reversible causes of MCI, there are no "easy fixes," and lifestyle modifications with dietary changes and enhanced physical and mental activity levels yield only modest results.

SUMMARY

MCI occurs along a continuum with normal cognition at one end of the continuum and dementia at the other. It is not always a precursor to Alzheimer disease and cognition may never progress beyond "mild impairment." One roadblock to earlier diagnosis and potential treatment is the lack of consistency with screening for MCI by physicians. Universal screening of certain age groups would be ideal, but is limited at this time owing to a lack of established guidelines, physician unawareness, and both time and financial constraints. However, once a diagnosis of MCI is made, it is important for the clinician to evaluate for reversible causes, particularly polypharmacy, obstructive sleep apnea, and depression, because treatment of these conditions can reverse or slow cognitive decline. Early diagnosis can be a gift to patients and families, because it allows time for getting legal and financial affairs in order, enables the patient to participate in shared decision making, and helps to establish plans for living arrangements, driving cessation, and so on, so that crisis situations can be avoided. At the present time, there are no pharmacologic treatments proven to slow or cure progression of MCI to dementia; nonetheless, there is evidence that lifestyle modifications including diet, exercise, and cognitive stimulation may be effective.

REFERENCES

1. Petersen RC, Smith GE, Waring SC, et al. Aging, memory and mild cognitive impairment. Int Psychogeriatr 1997;9(Suppl 1):65–9.
2. Sachdev PS, Blackner D, Blazer DG, et al. Classifying neurocognitive disorders: the DSM-5 approach. Nat Rev Neurol 2014;10(11):634–42.
3. American Psychiatric Association. Diagnostic and statistical manual of mental disorders. 5th edition. Arlington (VA): American Psychiatric Association; 2013.
4. Petersen RC, Morris JC. Mild cognitive impairment as a clinical entity and treatment target. Arch Neurol 2005;62(7):1160–3.
5. Stokin GB, Krell-Roesch J, Petersen RC, et al. Mild neurocognitive disorder: an old wine in a new bottle. Harv Rev Psychiatry 2015;23(5):368–76.
6. Petersen RC, Roberts RO, Knopman DS, et al. Prevalence of mild cognitive impairment is higher in men. The Mayo clinic study of aging. Neurology 2010; 75:889–97.
7. Ganguli M, Dodge HH, Shen C, et al. Mild cognitive impairment, amnestic type: an epidemiologic study. Neurology 2004;63:115–21.
8. Hanninen T, Hallikainen M, Tuomainen S, et al. Prevalence of mild cognitive impairment: a population-based study in elderly subjects. Acta Neurol Scand 2002;106:148–54.
9. Pandya SY, Clem MA, Silva LM, et al. Does mild cognitive impairment always lead to dementia? A review. J Neurol Sci 2016;369:57–62.
10. Roberts RO, Geda YE, Knopman DS, et al. The incidence of MCI differs by subtype and is higher in men. Neurology 2012;78:342–51.
11. Caselli RJ, Dueck AC, Osborne D, et al. Longitudinal modeling of age-related memory decline and the APOE epsilon4 effect. N Engl J Med 2009;361:255–63.
12. Ng TP, Feng L, Nyunt MS, et al. Metabolic syndrome and the risk of mild cognitive impairment and progression to dementia: follow-up of the Singapore Longitudinal Ageing Study Cohort. JAMA Neurol 2016;73(4):456–63.
13. Vassilaki M, Aakre JA, Cha RH, et al. Multimorbidity and risk of mild cognitive impairment. J Am Geriatr Soc 2015;63(9):1783–90.

14. Singh B, Mielke MM, Parsaik AK, et al. A prospective study of chronic obstructive pulmonary disease and the risk for mild cognitive impairment. JAMA Neurol 2014; 71:581–8.

15. Geda YE, Roberts RO, Mielke MM, et al. Baseline neuropsychiatric symptoms and the risk of incident mild cognitive impairment: a population-based study. Am J Psychiatry 2014;171:572–81.

16. Roberts RO, Knopman DS, Geda YE, et al. Association of diabetes with amnestic and nonamnestic mild cognitive impairment. Alzheimers Dement 2014;10:18–26.

17. Verghese J, LeValley A, Derby C, et al. Leisure activities and the risk of amnestic mild cognitive impairment in the elderly. Neurology 2006;66:821–7.

18. Geda YE, Roberts RO, Knopman DS, et al. Physical exercise, aging, and mild cognitive impairment: a population-based study. Arch Neurol 2010;67:80–6.

19. Han JW, Kim TH, Lee SB, et al. Predictive validity and diagnostic stability of mild cognitive impairment subtypes. Alzheimers Dement 2012;8(6):553–9.

20. Manly JJ, Tang MX, Schupf N, et al. Frequency and course of mild cognitive impairment in a multiethnic community. Ann Neurol 2008;63(4):494–506.

21. Ravaglia G, Forti P, Montesi F, et al. Mild cognitive impairment: epidemiology and dementia risk in an elderly Italian population. J Am Geriatr Soc 2008;56(1):51–8.

22. Artero S, Ancelin ML, Portet F, et al. Risk profiles for mild cognitive impairment and progression to dementia are gender specific. J Neurol Neurosurg Psychiatr 2008;79(9):979–84.

23. Sachdev PS, Lipnicki DM, Crawford J, et al. Factors predicting reversion from mild cognitive impairment to normal cognitive functioning: a population-based study. PLoS One 2013;8(3):e59649.

24. Mitchell AJ, Shiri-Feshki A. Rate of progression of mild cognitive impairment to dementia—meta-analysis of 41 robust inception cohort studies. Acta Psychiatr Scand 2009;119(4):252–65.

25. Roberts RO, Knopman DS, Mielke MM, et al. Higher risk of progression to dementia in mild cognitive impairment cases who revert to normal. Neurology 2014;82(4):317–25.

26. Morris JC. Mild cognitive impairment is early-stage Alzheimer disease: time to revise diagnostic criteria. Arch Neurol 2006;63:15–6.

27. Molano J, Boeve B, Ferman T, et al. Mild cognitive impairment associated with limbic and neocortical Lewy body disease: a clinicopathological study. Brain 2010;133:540–56.

28. Campbell N, Boustani M, Limbil T, et al. The cognitive impact of anticholinergics: a clinical review. Clin Interv Aging 2009;4:225–33.

29. Morley JE. Anticholinergic medications and cognition. J Am Med Dir Assoc 2011; 12(8):543.e1.

30. Elmstahl S, Widerstrom E. Orthostatic intolerance predicts mild cognitive impairment: incidence of mild cognitive impairment and dementia from the Swedish general population cohort good aging in Skane. Clin Interv Aging 2014;9:1993–2002.

31. Liu H, Gao S, Hall KS, et al. Optimal blood pressure for cognitive function: findings from an elderly African-American cohort study. J Am Geriatr Soc 2013;61(6): 875–81.

32. Johnson LA, Hall JR, O'Bryant SE. A depressive endophenotype of mild cognitive impairment and Alzheimer's disease. PLoS One 2013;8:1–8.

33. Modrego PJ, Ferrandez J. Depression in patients with mild cognitive impairment increases the risk of developing dementia of Alzheimer type: a prospective cohort study. Arch Neurol 2004;61:1290–3.

34. Van Boxtel MP, Menheere PP, Bekers O, et al. Thyroid function, depressed mood, and cognitive performance in older individuals: the Maastricht Aging Study. Psychoneuroendocrinology 2004;29(7):891–8.

35. Yaffe K, Falvey CM, Hamilton N, et al. Association between hypoglycemia and dementia in a biracial cohort of older adults with diabetes mellitus. JAMA Intern Med 2013;173(14):1300–6.

36. Bonetti F, Brombo G, Magon S, et al. Cognitive status according to homocysteine and B-group vitamins in elderly adults. J Am Geriatr Soc 2015;63(6):1158–63.

37. Chen LY, Agarwal SK, Norby FL, et al. Persistent but not paroxysmal atrial fibrillation is independently associated with lower cognitive function: ARIC Study. J Am Coll Cardiol 2016;67(100):1379–80.

38. Daulatzai MA. Evidence of neurodegeneration in obstructive sleep apnea: relationship between obstructive sleep apnea and cognitive dysfunction in the elderly. J Neurosci Res 2015;93(12):1778–94.

39. Cruz-Oliver DM, Malmstrom TK, Roegner M, et al. Cognitive deficit reversal as shown by changes in the veterans affairs Saint Louis University mental status (SLUMS) examination scores 7.5 years later. J Am Med Dir Assoc 2014;15(9): 687.e5-10.

40. Picascia M, Zangaglia R, Bernini S, et al. A review of cognitive impairment and differential diagnosis in idiopathic normal pressure hydrocephalus. Funct Neurol 2015;30(4):217–28.

41. Morley JE, Morris JC, Berg-Wegner M, et al. Brain health: the importance of recognizing cognitive impairment: an IAGG consensus conference. J Am Med Dir Assoc 2015;16(9):731–9.

42. Bradford A, Kunik ME, Schulz P, et al. Missed and delayed diagnosis of dementia in primary care: prevalence and contributing factors. Alzheimer Dis Assoc Disord 2009;23(4):306–14.

43. Tariq SH, Tumosa N, Chibnall JT, et al. Comparison of the Saint Louis University mental status examination and the mini-mental state examination for detecting dementia and mild neurocognitive disorder—a pilot study. Am J Geriatr Psychiatry 2006;14:900–10.

44. Malmstrom TK, Voss VB, Cruz-Oliver DM, et al. Rapid cognitive screen (RCS): a point-of-care screening for dementia and mild cognitive impairment. J Nutr Health Aging 2015;19:741–4.

45. Nasreddine ZS, Phillips NA, Bedirian V, et al. The Montreal Cognitive Assessment, MoCA: a brief screening tool for mild cognitive impairment. J Am Geriatr Soc 2005;53(4):695–9.

46. Yuan Y, Gu ZX, Wei WS. Fluorodeoxyglucose-positron-emission tomography, single-photon emission tomography, and structural MR imaging for prediction of rapid conversion to Alzheimer disease in patients with mild cognitive impairment: a meta-analysis. AJNR Am J Neuroradiol 2009;30:404–10.

47. Karow DS, McEvoy LK, Fennema-Notestine C, et al. Relative capability of MR imaging and FDG PET to depict changes associated with prodromal and early Alzheimer disease. Radiology 2010;256:932–42.

48. Wicklund M, Petersen RC. Emerging biomarkers in cognition. Clin Geriatr Med 2013;29(4):809–28.

49. Mattsson N, Zetterberg H, Hansson O, et al. CSF biomarkers and incipient Alzheimer disease in patients with mild cognitive impairment. JAMA 2009;302: 385–93.

50. Hansson O, Zetterberg H, Buchhave P, et al. Association between CSF biomarkers and incipient Alzheimer's disease in patients with mild cognitive impairment: a follow-up study. Lancet Neurol 2006;5:228–34.
51. Johnson KA, Minoshima S, Bohnen NI, et al. Appropriate use criteria for amyloid PET: a report of the amyloid imaging task force, the society of nuclear medicine and molecular imaging, and the Alzheimer's Association. Alzheimers Dement 2013;9:e1–16.
52. Jack CR, Wiste HJ, Vemuri P, et al. Brain beta-amyloid measures and magnetic resonance imaging atrophy both predict time-to-progression from mild cognitive impairment to Alzheimer's disease. Brain 2010;133:3336–48.
53. Ishii K. PET approaches for diagnosis of dementia. AJNR Am J Neuroradiol 2014; 35(11):2030–8.
54. Ganguli M, Fu B, Snitz BE, et al. Mild cognitive impairment: incidence and vascular risk factors in a population-based cohort. Neurology 2013;80(23): 2112–20.
55. Raschetti R, Albanese E, Vanacore N. Cholinesterase inhibitors in mild cognitive impairment: a systematic review of randomised trials. PLos Med 2007;4(11):e338.
56. Cooper C, Li R, Lyketsos C, et al. A systematic review of treatments for mild cognitive impairment. Br J Psychiatry 2013;203(3):255–64.
57. Petersen RC, Thomas RG, Grundman M. Vitamin E and donepezil for the treatment of mild cognitive impairment. N Engl J Med 2005;352(23):2379–88.
58. Naeini AM, Elmadfa I, Djazayery A, et al. The effect of antioxidant vitamins E and C on cognitive performance of the elderly with mild cognitive impairment in Isfahan, Iran: a double-blind, randomized, placebo-controlled trial. Eur J Nutr 2014;53(5):1255062.
59. Li MM, Yu JT, Wang HF, et al. Efficacy of vitamins B supplementation on mild cognitive impairment and Alzheimer's disease: a systematic review and meta-analysis. Curr Alzheimer Res 2014;11(9):844–52.
60. Snitz BE, O'Meara ES, Carlson MC, et al. Ginko biloba for preventing cognitive decline in older adults: a randomized trial. JAMA 2009;302(24):2663–70.
61. Krause D, Roupas P. Effect of vitamin intake on cognitive decline in older adults: evaluation of the evidence. J Nutr Health Aging 2015;19(7):745–53.
62. Cheng D, Kong H, Pang W, et al. B vitamin supplementation improves cognitive function in the middle aged and elderly with hyperhomocysteinemia. Nutr Neurosci 2016;19(10):461–6.
63. Solfrizzi V, Panza F. Mediterranean diet and cognitive decline. A lesson learned from the whole diet approach: what challenges lie ahead? J Alzheimers Dis 2014;39(2):283–6.
64. Singh B, Parsaik AK, Mielke MM, et al. Association of Mediterranean diet with mild cognitive impairment and Alzheimer's disease: a systematic review and meta-analysis. J Alzheimers Dis 2014;39(2):271–82.
65. Sofi F, Valecchi D, Bacci D, et al. Physical activity and risk of cognitive decline: a meta-analysis of prospective studies. J Intern Med 2011;269:107–17.
66. Gomez-Pinilla F, So V, Kesslak JP. Spatial learning and physical activity contribute to the induction of fibroblast growth factor: neural substrates for increased cognition associated with exercise. Neuroscience 1998;85:53–61.
67. Hall CB, Lipton RB, Sliwinski M, et al. Cognitive activities delay onset of memory decline in persons who develop dementia. Neurology 2009;73(5):356–61.
68. Aguirre E, Woods RT, Spector A, et al. Cognitive stimulation for dementia: a systematic review of the evidence of effectiveness from randomised controlled trials. Ageing Res Rev 2013;12(1):253–62.

Cognitive Frailty

Mechanisms, Tools to Measure, Prevention and Controversy

Bertrand Fougère, MD, PhD[a,b,*], Julien Delrieu, MD[a],
Natalia del Campo, PhD[a,c], Gaëlle Soriano[a],
Sandrine Sourdet, MD[a,b], Bruno Vellas, MD, PhD[a,b]

KEYWORDS

- Cognition • Cognitive frailty • Frailty • Mechanisms • Prevention

KEY POINTS

- Frailty has been linked to cognitive impairment.
- Shared mechanisms might include both shared subcellular pathophysiology (eg, cardiovascular risk factors, nutrition, hormonal changes, inflammation, accumulation of neurotoxic β-amyloid in the brain, nigral neuronal loss, lifestyle, and mental health issues).
- Effective screening and diagnostic tools exploring and identifying causes of frailty including cognitive status need to be developed.
- Multidomain interventions seem to be efficient in the prevention of cognitive frailty.
- Investigations and real randomized controlled trials are needed to improve appropriate treatment options for cognitive frailty.

INTRODUCTION

The increase in life expectancy is a global phenomenon, affecting developed and underdeveloped countries. Aging is the progressive and overall physiologic decline of the reserves of an organism, which decreases the ability to generate adaptive responses and sustain homeostasis. Given the difficulty in reversing aging's disabling cascades, it is important to act preventively with specifically tailored interventions against prodromal signs of disease and disability when these processes are still amenable to effective modification. Frailty is a pathologic aging process that is

Disclosure Statement: The authors have nothing to disclose.
[a] Gérontopôle, Centre Hospitalier Universitaire de Toulouse, Toulouse, France; [b] Inserm UMR1027, Université de Toulouse III Paul Sabatier, Toulouse, France; [c] Centre of Exellence in Neurodegeneration, Centre Hospitalier Universitaire de Toulouse, Toulouse, France
* Corresponding author. Institut du Vieillissement, Gérontopôle, Université Toulouse III Paul Sabatier, 37 Allées Jules Guesde, Toulouse 31000, France.
E-mail address: b.fougere@gmail.com

reversible and occurs at an intermediate stage between age-related diseases and a poor prognosis, such as disability or death.[1–4] This syndrome is triggering considerable attention not only in clinics and research, but also among public health authorities.[1] Most of the available definitions have privileged the physical dimension of the frailty syndrome, mostly relying on symptoms and signs like weight loss, muscle weakness, slow gait speed, and sedentary behavior.[5] Nevertheless, a growing body of evidence suggests that other factors (eg, nutrition,[6] mental health,[7] and cognition[8]) may also influence the frailty status of the older individual. Based on different pathogeneses, frailty can be divided into physical frailty, cognitive frailty, and psychosocial frailty.[9,10] Cognitive frailty is increasingly recognized as a fundamental determinant of the individual's vulnerability and resilience to stressors.[11] Several investigators have also supported the idea that individuals who manifest both cognitive and motor deficits might have a greater burden of a shared underlying pathologic condition. They introduced a new idea that they refer to as *motoric cognitive risk* syndrome,[12–14] a concept closely connected with cognitive frailty. This report refines the framework for the definition and mechanisms of cognitive frailty and relevant screening tools. Furthermore, we explore the possible prevention of the cognitive frailty progression. Finally, we comment on the controversy that exists in the field.

THE COGNITIVE FRAILTY APPROACH
The Proposed Definition of Cognitive Frailty

In 2001, the term *cognitive frailty* was used by Paganini-Hill and colleagues[15] in a study on Clock Drawing Test (CDT) performance and its association with potential protective and risk factors for Alzheimer's disease (AD) in an older cohort. In 2006, cognitive frailty was proposed by Panza and colleagues[16] when these authors examined the risks of decreased cognitive functions modulated by vascular factors. Subsequent studies found that physical factors and cognition are crucial elements in predicting risk of death.[10,16,17] In 2013, a consensus on the definition of cognitive frailty was reached by an international consensus group (the International Academy on Nutrition and Aging and the International Association of Gerontology and Geriatrics).[18] The panel defined cognitive frailty as a syndrome in older adults with evidence of both physical frailty and cognitive impairment without a clinical diagnosis of AD or another dementia (Clinical Dementia Rating score [CDR] = 0.5).[18] This finding implies that cognitive frailty is a form of pathologic brain aging and a precursor to neurodegenerative processes. With this definition, physical frailty and cognition are associated; however, the causal links between physical frailty and cognitive impairment are not clear.

The History of the Link Between Frailty and Cognitive Impairment

Based on the different domains and the multidimensional nature of frailty, this geriatric syndrome can be divided into physical frailty, cognitive frailty, and psychosocial frailty,[10,19] with this last definition suggesting that frailty may also affect quality of life and social connectivity.[20] In particular, in 2001, the term *cognitive frailty* was incidentally used by Paganini-Hill and colleagues.[15] In 2006, this clinical label was first used to indicate a particular state of cognitive vulnerability in mild cognitive impairment (MCI) and other similar clinical entities exposed to the risk modulated by vascular factors with a subsequent increased progression to dementia, particularly vascular dementia.[16] Thus, cognition plays an important role in the manifestation of the frailty syndrome. In this context, some investigators have proposed the addition of a cognitive assessment within the operational definitions of frailty. For example, Rockwood and colleagues[21–23] consider frailty as a cumulative index of health deficits, including cognitive impairment, and developed and validate the so-called Frailty Index. Cognitive impairment has been independently associated with several adverse outcomes (eg, falls, hospitalization, and mortality), even when specific conditions (eg, dementia and MCI) were considered.[24] Cross-sectional studies document high rates of cognitive impairment in frail compared with robust older persons, being observed in nearly 20% of frail individuals living in the community[25] (**Table 1**). Consistently, longitudinal studies repeatedly reported that physical frailty predicts the onset of future cognitive decline and incident dementia[8] (see **Table 1**). The reciprocal association (ie, cognitive impairment predicts future frailty) has also been observed.[26] In addition to these epidemiologic evidences, various studies suggest that there are multiple interrelated mechanisms that may mediate these associations, including chronic inflammation, nutritional patterns, vascular disease, depression, and endocrine deficiencies.[27]

The Relationship Between Frailty and Cognition

Many pathologic processes contribute to cognitive impairment, leading to several possible avenues for dementia prevention. Age is consistently reported as the most important independent risk factor for cognitive impairment and dementia, and so it is likely that many of the age-associated processes that lead to frailty in older people are also responsible for brain aging and consequent cognitive decline. The place of cognitive impairment in a definition of frailty has been widely debated. The model by Fried and colleagues[5] describes a wasting syndrome, with weight loss and negative energy balance as important elements and does not include cognitive function in its definition, whereas the model by Rockwood and colleagues[21–23] allows poor cognition to be included as one of the possible deficits. A review of frailty measures found that the most commonly included components in an operational definition of frailty were physical function, gait, speed, and cognition, with cognition being included in 50% of the definitions.[28,29] On the other hand, statistical analyses on these proposed components of frailty suggest that, although physical activity, mobility, energy, strength, and mood aggregate are highly correlated, cognition does not correlate strongly with these other components and, therefore, may not be part of the frailty syndrome.[30,31] It seems most useful, therefore, to treat frailty and cognitive impairment as related but distinct concepts that frequently co-occur (**Fig. 1**).

THE MECHANISMS OF COGNITIVE FRAILTY

Numerous studies found that multiple risk factors that cause cognitive impairment are also associated with the development and worsening of physical frailty in older individuals.[8,18,24] The risk factors include cardiovascular events (eg, diabetes, dyslipidemia, hypertension), nutritional deficiencies (eg, malnutrition, vitamin D deficiency), hormonal imbalance (eg, reduced testosterone, insulin resistance), inflammation, accumulation of neurotoxic β-amyloid (Aβ) in the brain, nigral neuronal loss, lifestyle, and mental health issues[8,18,24] (**Fig. 2**).

Cardiovascular Risk Factors

Cardiovascular risk factors and common vascular diseases have been related to both frailty[32] and cognitive impairment.[16] In fact, several studies found that comorbidities like congestive heart failure, myocardial infarction, peripheral arterial diseases, diabetes mellitus, and hypertension increased the risk for frailty.[32,33] The association between physical frailty and increased risk of incident cognitive impairment may be linked to an underlying increased risk of stroke and cerebrovascular disease. In

Table 1
Recent studies on the association between frailty and cognitive function

Study and Year	Type of RCT	Participants	Tools Used	Findings
Alencar et al,[106] 2013	Longitudinal studies	N = 207 1 y	Physical frailty phenotype assessed with the CHS criteria. Cognitive function and dementia evaluated with MMSE and CDR.	Frailty was associated with a subsequent decline in cognitive function when measured using the MMSE. No statistically significant differences among the different classifications of frailty were detected regarding the decline in cognitive function when assessed using the CDR.
Ferrer et al,[107] 2013	Cross-sectional studies	N = 273	Physical frailty phenotype operalizionated with the CHS criteria. Cognitive function was evaluated with MMSE.	The overall prevalence of frailty and cognitive impairment and frailty and dementia combined was 55.4%, and 26.8%, respectively.
Forti et al,[108] 2014	Longitudinal studies	N = 766 7 y	Physical frailty phenotype operalizionated with SOF index. Cognitive function assessed with CDT.	The CDT may predict the mortality risk independently of the physical phenotype of frailty.
Gray et al,[109] 2013	Longitudinal studies	N = 2619 6.5 y	Physical frailty phenotype operalizionated with the CHS criteria. Diagnosis of dementia according to the DSM-IV, diagnosis of possible and probable AD according to NINCDS-ADRDA criteria.	Frailty was associated with higher risk of developing non-AD dementia but not AD.
Han et al,[110] 2014	Cross-sectional studies	N = 10,388	Physical frailty phenotype operalizionated with the CHS criteria. Cognitive function was assessed using MMSE.	Frail subjects showed a higher percentage of cognitive impairment, with some gender differences. Cognitive impairment was associated with a higher likelihood of frailty in community-dwelling older men and women.
Kulmala et al,[111] 2014	Cross-sectional studies	N = 654	Physical frailty phenotype operalizionated with the CHS criteria. Diagnosis of dementia, AD, and VaD according to the DSM-IV criteria and cognitive impairment evaluated with MMSE.	Frail persons were almost 8 times more likely to have cognitive impairment, 8 times more likely to have some kind of dementia, almost 6 times more likely to have VaD, and more than 4 times more likely to have AD than persons who were robust.

Study	Study type	N	Methods	Findings
Lee et al,[112] 2014	Longitudinal studies	N = 3018 2 y	Frailty phenotype operalizionated with the CHS criteria. Cognitive function was evaluated with MMSE.	Among prefrail participants, hospitalizations, older age, previous stroke, lower cognition, and osteoarthritis were risk factors associated with worsening to frail state or less improvement to robust state.
McGough et al,[113] 2013	Cross-sectional studies	N = 201	Physical frailty dimensions adapted from the CHS criteria. Severity of cognitive impairment was measured with the ADAS-Cog. Cognitive functions were evaluated with TMT-A, TMT-B, WMS-R Logical Memory, and the delayed Word Recall subitem of the ADAS-Cog.	Lower performance on dimensions of physical frailty was associated with worse performance on the ADAS-Cog. In particular, slower usual gait speed was associated with elevated severity of cognitive impairment and worse performance within all dimensions of memory, attention, and executive function.
Montero-Odasso et al,[114] 2016	Longitudinal studies	N = 252	Frailty was defined using validated phenotypic criteria. Cognition was assessed using the Montreal Cognitive Assessment. Gait was assessed using an electronic walkway.	Frailty participants had a higher prevalence of cognitive impairment compared with those without frailty but not significant risk to incident dementia. Cognitive frailty increased incident rate but not risk for progression to dementia. The combination of slow gait and cognitive impairment posed the highest risk for progression to dementia.
Rolfson et al,[115] 2013	Cross-sectional studies	N = 388	Frailty was defined with the CHS criteria, the EFS, and a frailty index. Cognitive function was assessed using MMSE and a test of visuomotor speed.	A relationship independent of the MMSE score was only demonstrated in the frailty index.
Runzer-Colmenares et al,[116] 2014	Cross-sectional studies	N = 311	Physical frailty phenotype operalizionated with the CHS criteria. Cognitive function was assessed with the CDT.	Frail subjects showed a higher percentage of cognitive impairment (41.9%), although cognitive function was not significantly associated with frailty.
Sampson et al,[117] 2013	Longitudinal studies	N = 616 1 y	Waterlow Scale, a frailty marker, evaluating the risk of pressure sores. Cognitive function assessed with MMSE, and	People with dementia had half the survival time of those without dementia. The effect of dementia on mortality was reduced after adjustment, particularly by the Waterlow score.

(continued on next page)

Table 1
(continued)

Study and Year	Type of RCT	Participants	Tools Used	Findings
			diagnosis of dementia according to the DSM-IV criteria.	
Schoufour et al,[118] 2014	Cross-sectional studies	N = 1050	Frailty was defined with a frailty index. Intellectual quotient scores, Vineland scores, and social emotional development were used to determine the level of cognitive disabilities.	The least frail group was characterized by the absence of mobility and physical fitness limitations, relative independence, fewer specific medical problems, and fewer signs of depression/dementia.
Shimada et al,[119] 2013	Cross-sectional studies	N = 5104	Physical frailty phenotype operalizionated slightly modifying the CHS criteria. MCI diagnosed according to international consensus criteria.	The overall prevalence of frailty, MCI, and frailty and MCI combined was 11.3%, 18.8%, and 2.7%, respectively. A significant relationship between frailty and MCI was also found.
Solfrizzi et al,[36] 2013	Longitudinal studies	N = 2581 3.5 y	Physical frailty phenotype operalizionated slightly modifying the CHS criteria. Diagnosis of dementia according to the DSM-III-R, NINCDS-ADRDA, and ICD-10 criteria.	Frailty syndrome was associated with a significantly increased risk of overall dementia and, in particular, VaD, whereas the risk of AD or other types of dementia did not significantly change in frail individuals compared with subjects without frailty syndrome.
Sourial et al,[120] 2013	Longitudinal studies	N = 3447 6 y	Seven frailty markers (cognition, energy, mobility, mood, nutrition, physical activity, and strength)	The "best model" in each cohort was found to be a model including between 5 and 7 frailty markers including cognition, mobility, nutrition, physical activity, and strength.

Abbreviations: ADAS-Cog, Alzheimer's Disease Assessment Scale-Cognitive Subscale; CHS, cardiovascular health study; DSM-III-R, Diagnostic and Statistical Manual of Mental Disorders-III revised; DSM-IV, Diagnostic and Statistical Manual of Mental Disorders-IV; EFS, Edmonton frail scale; ICD-10, International Statistical Classification of Diseases and Related Health Problems, 10th revision; NINCDS-ADRDA, National Institute of Neurological and Communicative Disorders and Stroke–Alzheimer's Disease and Related Disorders Association; SOF, study of osteoporotic fractures; VaD, vascular dementia; WMS-R, Wechsler memory scale revised.
Data from Refs.[36,106–120]

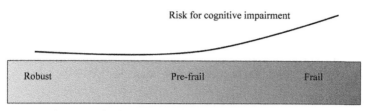

Fig. 1. Association between frailty and cognitive impairment.

fact, findings from the Cardiovascular Health Survey suggested that physical frailty was clearly related to subclinical vascular biomarkers and higher degree of infarctlike lesions in the brain.[34] Moreover, longitudinal population-based studies also suggested physical frailty as a prodromal stage of vascular dementia.[35,36] Finally, sarcopenia, an age-related decline in skeletal muscle mass and muscle function and a reliable marker of frailty, may be accelerated by comorbid conditions including vascular diseases such as congestive heart failure and peripheral arterial diseases.[37] Sarcopenia could worsen prognosis of neurodegenerative diseases including AD, and a link also exists between sarcopenia and cognitive decline.[38]

Nutrition

Nutrition may also play a role in the link between cognition and frailty because of the biological and behavioral effects of diet.[39] Sarcopenia is thought to be strongly associated with development of frailty and cognitive impairment, perhaps owing to oxidative stress.[38,40] Adherence to a Mediterranean diet, high in antioxidants, has been linked to lower frailty and better cognitive function.[40,41] In a recent randomized controlled trial (RCT) with a 6.5-year follow-up, nutritional intervention with a Mediterranean diet enhanced with extra-virgin olive oil or mixed nuts seemed to improve

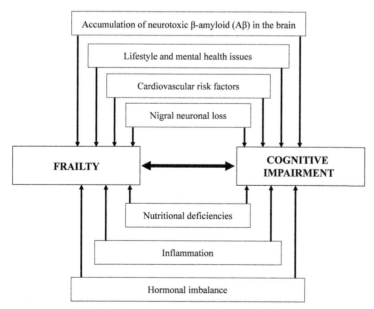

Fig. 2. Mechanisms underlying the observed link between frailty and cognitive impairment.

global cognition after adjustment for possible confounders.[42] Moreover, in a cross-sectional population-based study, higher adherence to a Mediterranean diet was inversely linked to prevalence of frailty.[43] Taken together, these findings may suggest a long-term effect of a Mediterranean diet both on frailty and cognitive function in older age even if other studies showed effects more nuanced.[44,45]

Hormonal Changes

Reviews suggest that reduced testosterone and other androgen hormones may be involved in the development of frailty and cognitive decline.[46,47] Testosterone is thought to have protective effects on cognition through its promotion of synaptic plasticity in the hippocampus and its regulation of the accumulation of Aβ protein.[46] Furthermore, age-related depletion of testosterone is thought to be associated with declining muscle mass, an important factor in the development of frailty.[47] It is thus possible that reduced testosterone may be a mediator in this relationship or common underlying factor to both frailty and cognitive decline.

Inflammation

The mechanisms of inflammation in cognitive impairment have already been described.[48,49] Increased serum concentrations of interleukin (IL)-8 are associated with poor performance in memory and speed domains and in motor function.[50] IL-6 and C-reactive protein are also prospectively associated with cognitive decline in older subjects.[51] On the other hand, immune system changes and inflammation are also associated with frailty. Data considering the effect of inflammation on frailty suggest that the inflammatory processes triggered by some cytokines, especially IL-6, tumor necrosis factor-α and other inflammatory proteins are associated in the older subject with increased risk of morbidity and mortality, and cohort studies indicate tumor necrosis factor-α and IL-6 levels as markers of frailty.[52–55] Consequently, the inflammatory process seems to have a role in the development of both frailty and cognitive impairment.[40]

Accumulation of Neurotoxic β-Amyloid in the Brain

Aβ pathology in the brain causes slowing of gait speed, by a direct neurotoxic effect, by accelerating tau deposition or by other mechanisms. According to the prevailing amyloid cascade hypothesis, Aβ leads to the formation of tau tangles, which are primarily responsible for local synaptic dysfunction, neurodegeneration, and neuronal loss.[56,57] Consistent with this view, Aβ-induced tau tangles but not amyloid per se would be expected to have local neurotoxic effects with implications for the regulation of motor and sensorimotor circuits. However, there are reports of in vitro and animal studies that Aβ, independent of tau tangles, disrupts synaptic function in the immediate vicinity of Aβ plaques altering the organization of related neural networks,[58–60] supporting the notion that Aβ toxicity can also cause neuronal dysfunction. A study found a significant association between gait speed, marker of the frailty phenotype, and brain Aβ (measured with amyloid PET) in the posterior and anterior putamen, the occipital cortex, precuneus, and anterior cingulate, independent of age, ApoE genotype, and disease stage.[61] Another study speculated that accumulation of AD pathology in brain regions that subserve cognition could affect components of frailty by impairing neural systems involved in the planning and monitoring of even simple movements.[62]

Nigral Neuronal Loss

The substantia nigra represents a structural component of neural reserve that contributes to brain reserve capacity.[63] In a meta-analysis, neuronal density in the locus ceruleus, dorsal raphe nucleus, and substantia nigra was reduced in AD.[64] A study found that not only AD conditions but also several cerebrovascular conditions and nigral neuronal loss, a common finding in Parkinson disease, were associated with the rate of progression of physical frailty in community-dwelling older adults. These associations were robust and unchanged after controlling for baseline chronic health conditions and disability, excluding cases of Parkinson disease, and did not vary by dementia status.[65]

Lifestyle and Mental Health Issues

Depression is both a risk factor for and a consequence of frailty.[66,67] Depression is also known to affect cognitive function.[68]This finding suggests that one mechanism underlying the link between frailty and cognition may be owing to psychological factors such as mood. Recently, a study found that participants with vascular depression at baseline were significantly more likely to have frailty.[67] Fifty-five percent of participants with vascular depression became frail within 4 years compared with 35% of participants with a high cerebrovascular burden alone and 25% of participants with neither. This finding suggests that in addition to the aforementioned link with vascular events, the interaction between the vascular burden and mood effects of depression is an important consideration in understanding frailty. In parallel, several studies suggested that lifestyle factors have a significant impact on how well people age. For example, Fratiglioni and colleagues[69] reported that 3 lifestyle factors can play a significant role in slowing the rate of cognitive decline and preventing dementia: a socially integrated network, cognitive leisure activity, and regular physical activity. In this review and others,[70,71] it is argued that out of these lifestyle factors, physical activity has the most support as protective against the deleterious effects of age on health and cognition.

THE TOOLS TO MEASURE COGNITIVE FRAILTY

To design effective interventions for cognitive frailty, effective screening and diagnostic tools allowing the exploration and identification of the causes underlying frailty, including cognitive status, need to be developed. This tool gives us the opportunity to better detect the possible future health trajectories that a frail person with cognitive impairment will follow. Consequently, this differentiation allows the design of better personalized preventive or therapeutic interventions.

Possible biomarkers, clinical markers, and imaging techniques are used to characterize and eventually predict distinct age trajectories. To identify cognitive frailty, the panel suggested that all the frail subjects should perform a comprehensive cognitive assessment exploring memory performance and other cognitive functions (ie, executive functions). The objective was to exclude the diagnosis of AD. The International Psychogeriatric Association survey found 20 brief cognitive instruments that respondents used in clinical practice chosen for "effectiveness," "ease of administration," and "familiarity."[72] The Mini-Mental State Examination (MMSE)[73] was the most common, followed by the CDT.[74] Other cognitive tests and instruments to identify cognitive frailty could be suggested: Frontal Assessment Battery,[75] the 5 words test,[76] Free and Cued Selective Reminding Test,[77] Trail Making Test (TMT) Parts A and B,[78] Wechsler Adult Intelligence Scale revised, and coding and verbal fluencies as diagnosis tests.[79] The Mattis Dementia Rating Scale[80] could also be proposed. Biomarkers of preclinical AD include the following: markers of Aβ accumulation, such as the level of amyloid-β42 in cerebrospinal fluid, and PET amyloid imaging; markers of neurodegeneration or neuronal injury, including the level of tau and phosphorylated tau protein in cerebrospinal fluid; ^{18}F-fluorodeoxyglucose PET functional imaging or functional MRI; and nerve degeneration or damage, such as that found by the MRI–based detection of hippocampus atrophy or cortical thinning. The assessment of nigral neuronal loss and white matter lesions could be also useful in his context. Based on various combinations of Aβ aggregation, nerve degeneration, and the subtle reduction of cognitive function, preclinical AD can be divided into 4 stages.[81] In addition, homozygous ApoE ε4 is a useful biomarker for late-onset familial and sporadic AD patients.

In parallel, usual physical frailty markers (such as weight loss and gait speed) should be assessed in persons exhibiting a cognitive decline. Based on the mechanisms of frailty, including those of phenotypic defect accumulation and the aggregation of multifunctional domains, various frailty screening techniques have been indicated.[28,82,83] Among these, Fried's phenotypic physiology-based screening is being preferentially used for frailty research,[5] whereas scales for frailty resulting from defect accumulation are more suitable for health management, such as predicting whether an elderly individual requires hospitalization.[22] Some markers may be able to capture well the risk of both future physical and cognitive decline, such as inflammatory biomarkers (C-reactive protein, IL-6).[53,84–86] However, biomarkers predictive of both types of decline may not be particularly useful in differentiating whether a person is at higher risk of a future physical rather than a cognitive decline and vice versa.

THE PREVENTION OF COGNITIVE FRAILTY

For the older subjects, primary preventive intervention includes the promotion of physical activities, cognitive stimulation, exercise and a healthy diet (a Mediterranean diet), the cessation of smoking, promoting emotional recovery, engaging in an active and socially integrated lifestyle, an ideal amount of daily sleep, the maintenance of a proper body weight, and metabolic control (including the control of dyslipidemia, diabetes, and blood pressure).[28,87] At this stage, secondary prevention strategies for cognitive impairment and physical frailty are suggested. For the older subjects with potential cognitive frailty, secondary prevention is required, which comprises a geriatric assessment determining the cause of cognitive frailty and an evidence-based, medicinal, individualized multimodal intervention. Other measures, such as drug treatment for chronic diseases, fall prevention, and exercise and nutrition support, which target physical, nutritional, cognitive, and psychological domains, may delay the progression and secondary occurrence of cognitive frailty related adverse outcomes.[1,18,28,87] In fact, a multidomain intervention seems to be efficient in the prevention of cognitive frailty.

Although evidence on interventions in frailty coupled with cognitive decline is limited, a small number of studies point to the cognitive benefits of physical activity. In 2010, a review found that physical activity protected against both sarcopenia and cognitive decline in experimental training trials and in observational studies.[88] A study for frailty and cognitive decline found that an aerobic exercise and strength training program for frail older adults improved scores in functional capacity and physical endurance, cognition, and quality of life.[89] The significant improvements in cognition were caused by increased scores in measures of working memory, processing speed, and executive function.

COGNITIVE FRAILTY CONTROVERSY

The concept of cognitive frailty has been proposed for framing the growing and consistent evidence linking physical and cognitive decline in older persons within recognizable and discriminative standards. However, a new clinical entity should be clearly defined from the previous entities defining cognitive impairment in older persons. Thus, it is also difficult to distinguish the difference between cognitive frailty and cognitive reserve. *Cognitive reserve* refers to the capacity of a given individual to resist cognitive impairment or decline. Educational level and prior cognitive abilities are important determinants of cognitive reserve.[90–92] Cognitive reserve has been linked with resilience of brain function and structure in the presence of disease, injury, or other factors that alter physiologic functioning.[93]

A major controversial point regarding the definition of cognitive frailty is reversible cognitive impairment (CDR = 0.5), which can be confusing. It was proposed that a CDR value of 0.5 was equivalent to the MCI stage.[94,95] Some MCI patients have symptoms that are reversible and can recover to regain normal cognitive function. The cognitive functions of other patients may even be stable and not change throughout the remainder of their lives. However, more MCI patients exhibit an irreversible, progressive reduction in cognition.[96–98]

Several studies addressed the relationship between frailty and cognition. Delrieu and colleagues[99] attempted to characterize the "cognitive frailty" entity in a cohort of 1617 subjects enrolled in Multidomain Alzheimer Disease Preventive Trial (MAPT). Their cognitive frailty sample represented 22% of the population. However, there are no RCTs found in the field "cognitive frailty," underlining the scarcity of available evidence.[100] In fact, RCTs could provide useful information concerning the possibility of positively affecting the frailty syndrome by acting on cognition and improving cognition by targeting the physical components of frailty. These studies may provide key information to help characterize cognitive frailty and its underlying mechanisms and its reversibility. Furthermore, several RCTs were recently conducted to investigate the efficacy of physical interventions in improving cognitive functioning in healthy elderly individuals,[101,102] and other RCTs evaluated the effectiveness of multidomain interventions in preventing cognitive decline in older adults at risk of dementia.[103,104] However, no study has specifically targeted populations of cognitive frail older persons. Thus, there is currently a lack of sensitive and specific methods to detect cognitive frailty at the clinical level. Several investigators stress the importance of establishing a useful clinical entity because of its possible reversibility.[105] It is clear that longitudinal studies that incorporate cognition, physical frailty, and psychological constructs such as depression are needed.

SUMMARY

Because of the population, the burden of aging-related conditions such as dementia and frailty is increasing. Available data corroborate the clear association between frailty and cognitive impairment via common underlying mechanisms including vascular and hormonal changes, nutrient deficiencies, and inflammation. The benefits of understanding the relationship between cognition and frailty are 2-fold. First, frail individuals are likely to be at high risk of cognitive impairment and vice versa. Second, understanding the link between frailty and cognition may lead to new interventions for the prevention and management of both conditions. Thus, cognitive frailty represents a window of opportunity for the prevention of adverse outcomes owing to aging, but important points remain to be clarified. In this context, further investigations and real longitudinal RCTs are needed to identify the common underlying mechanisms to improve appropriate treatment options for both conditions.

REFERENCES

1. Morley JE, Vellas B, van Kan GA, et al. Frailty consensus: a call to action. J Am Med Dir Assoc 2013;14(6):392–7.

2. Clegg A, Barber S, Young J, et al. The Home-based Older People's Exercise (HOPE) trial: a pilot randomised controlled trial of a home-based exercise intervention for older people with frailty. Age Ageing 2014;43(5):687–95.
3. Dorner TE, Lackinger C, Haider S, et al. Nutritional intervention and physical training in malnourished frail community-dwelling elderly persons carried out by trained lay "buddies": study protocol of a randomized controlled trial. BMC Public Health 2013;13:1232.
4. Tavassoli N, Guyonnet S, Abellan Van Kan G, et al. Description of 1,108 older patients referred by their physician to the "geriatric frailty clinic (G.F.C) for assessment of frailty and prevention of disability" at the gerontopole. J Nutr Health Aging 2014;18(5):457–64.
5. Fried LP, Tangen CM, Walston J, et al. Frailty in older adults: evidence for a phenotype. J Gerontol A Biol Sci Med Sci 2001;56(3):M146–56.
6. Kelaiditi E, van Kan GA, Cesari M. Frailty: role of nutrition and exercise. Curr Opin Clin Nutr Metab Care 2014;17(1):32–9.
7. Brown PJ, Roose SP, Fieo R, et al. Frailty and depression in older adults: a high-risk clinical population. Am J Geriatr Psychiatry 2014;22(11):1083–95.
8. Robertson DA, Savva GM, Kenny RA. Frailty and cognitive impairment–a review of the evidence and causal mechanisms. Ageing Res Rev 2013;12(4):840–51.
9. Malmstrom TK, Morley JE. Frailty and cognition: linking two common syndromes in older persons. J Nutr Health Aging 2013;17(9):723–5.
10. Panza F, Solfrizzi V, Frisardi V, et al. Different models of frailty in predementia and dementia syndromes. J Nutr Health Aging 2011;15(8):711–9.
11. Canevelli M, Troili F, Bruno G. Reasoning about frailty in neurology: neurobiological correlates and clinical perspectives. J Frailty Aging 2014;3(1):18–20.
12. Hausdorff JM, Buchman AS. What links gait speed and MCI with dementia? A fresh look at the association between motor and cognitive function. J Gerontol A Biol Sci Med Sci 2013;68(4):409–11.
13. Verghese J, Annweiler C, Ayers E, et al. Motoric cognitive risk syndrome: multi-country prevalence and dementia risk. Neurology 2014;83(8):718–26.
14. Camicioli R, Howieson D, Oken B, et al. Motor slowing precedes cognitive impairment in the oldest old. Neurology 1998;50(5):1496–8.
15. Paganini-Hill A, Clark LJ, Henderson VW, et al. Clock drawing: analysis in a retirement community. J Am Geriatr Soc 2001;49(7):941–7.
16. Panza F, D'Introno A, Colacicco AM, et al. Cognitive frailty: predementia syndrome and vascular risk factors. Neurobiol Aging 2006;27(7):933–40.
17. Pilotto A, Rengo F, Marchionni N, et al. Comparing the prognostic accuracy for all-cause mortality of frailty instruments: a multicentre 1-year follow-up in hospitalized older patients. PLoS One 2012;7(1):e29090.
18. Kelaiditi E, Cesari M, Canevelli M, et al. Cognitive frailty: rational and definition from an (I.A.N.A./I.A.G.G.) international consensus group. J Nutr Health Aging 2013;17(9):726–34.
19. Malmstrom TK, Morley JE. The frail brain. J Am Med Dir Assoc 2013;14(7): 453–5.
20. Langlois F, Vu TTM, Kergoat M-J, et al. The multiple dimensions of frailty: physical capacity, cognition, and quality of life. Int Psychogeriatr 2012;24(9): 1429–36.
21. Rockwood K, Song X, MacKnight C, et al. A global clinical measure of fitness and frailty in elderly people. CMAJ 2005;173(5):489–95.
22. Rockwood K, Mitnitski A. Frailty in relation to the accumulation of deficits. J Gerontol A Biol Sci Med Sci 2007;62(7):722–7.

23. Searle SD, Mitnitski A, Gahbauer EA, et al. A standard procedure for creating a frailty index. BMC Geriatr 2008;8:24.

24. Houles M, Canevelli M, Abellan Van Kan G. Frailty and cognition. J Frailty Aging 2012;1(2):56–63.

25. Avila-Funes JA, Amieva H, Barberger-Gateau P, et al. Cognitive impairment improves the predictive validity of the phenotype of frailty for adverse health outcomes: the three-city study. J Am Geriatr Soc 2009;57(3):453–61.

26. Raji MA, Al Snih S, Ostir GV, et al. Cognitive status and future risk of frailty in older Mexican Americans. J Gerontol A Biol Sci Med Sci 2010;65(11):1228–34.

27. Shah R. The role of nutrition and diet in Alzheimer disease: a systematic review. J Am Med Dir Assoc 2013;14(6):398–402.

28. Sternberg SA, Wershof Schwartz A, Karunananthan S, et al. The identification of frailty: a systematic literature review. J Am Geriatr Soc 2011;59(11):2129–38.

29. Dent E, Kowal P, Hoogendijk EO. Frailty measurement in research and clinical practice: a review. Eur J Intern Med 2016;31:3–10.

30. Sourial N, Bergman H, Karunananthan S, et al. Contribution of frailty markers in explaining differences among individuals in five samples of older persons. J Gerontol A Biol Sci Med Sci 2012;67(11):1197–204.

31. Sourial N, Wolfson C, Bergman H, et al. A correspondence analysis revealed frailty deficits aggregate and are multidimensional. J Clin Epidemiol 2010; 63(6):647–54.

32. Afilalo J, Karunananthan S, Eisenberg MJ, et al. Role of frailty in patients with cardiovascular disease. Am J Cardiol 2009;103(11):1616–21.

33. Lee JSW, Auyeung T-W, Leung J, et al. Physical frailty in older adults is associated with metabolic and atherosclerotic risk factors and cognitive impairment independent of muscle mass. J Nutr Health Aging 2011;15(10):857–62.

34. Newman AB, Gottdiener JS, Mcburnie MA, et al. Associations of subclinical cardiovascular disease with frailty. J Gerontol A Biol Sci Med Sci 2001;56(3): M158–66.

35. Avila-Funes JA, Carcaillon L, Helmer C, et al. Is frailty a prodromal stage of vascular dementia? Results from the Three-City Study. J Am Geriatr Soc 2012; 60(9):1708–12.

36. Solfrizzi V, Scafato E, Frisardi V, et al. Frailty syndrome and the risk of vascular dementia: the Italian Longitudinal Study on Aging. Alzheimers Dement 2013; 9(2):113–22.

37. Buford TW, Anton SD, Judge AR, et al. Models of accelerated sarcopenia: critical pieces for solving the puzzle of age-related muscle atrophy. Ageing Res Rev 2010;9(4):369–83.

38. Nourhashémi F, Andrieu S, Gillette-Guyonnet S, et al. Is there a relationship between fat-free soft tissue mass and low cognitive function? Results from a study of 7,105 women. J Am Geriatr Soc 2002;50(11):1796–801.

39. Khater MS, Abouelezz NF. Nutritional status in older adults with mild cognitive impairment living in elderly homes in Cairo, Egypt. J Nutr Health Aging 2011; 15(2):104–8.

40. Mulero J, Zafrilla P, Martinez-Cacha A. Oxidative stress, frailty and cognitive decline. J Nutr Health Aging 2011;15(9):756–60.

41. Talegawkar SA, Bandinelli S, Bandeen-Roche K, et al. A higher adherence to a Mediterranean-style diet is inversely associated with the development of frailty in community-dwelling elderly men and women. J Nutr 2012;142(12):2161–6.

42. Martínez-Lapiscina EH, Clavero P, Toledo E, et al. Mediterranean diet improves cognition: the PREDIMED-NAVARRA randomised trial. J Neurol Neurosurg Psychiatry 2013;84(12):1318–25.

43. Bollwein J, Diekmann R, Kaiser MJ, et al. Dietary quality is related to frailty in community-dwelling older adults. J Gerontol A Biol Sci Med Sci 2013;68(4):483–9.

44. Manal B, Suzana S, Singh DKA. Nutrition and frailty: a review of clinical intervention studies. J Frailty Aging 2015;4(2):100–6.

45. Vandewoude M, Barberger-Gateau P, Cederholm T, et al. Healthy brain ageing and cognition: nutritional factors. Eur Geriatr Med 2016;7(1):77–85.

46. Maggio M, Dall'Aglio E, Lauretani F, et al. The hormonal pathway to cognitive impairment in older men. J Nutr Health Aging 2012;16(1):40–54.

47. Muller M, Grobbee DE, Thijssen JHH, et al. Sex hormones and male health: effects on components of the frailty syndrome. Trends Endocrinol Metab 2003;14(6):289–96.

48. Aktas O, Ullrich O, Infante-Duarte C, et al. Neuronal damage in brain inflammation. Arch Neurol 2007;64(2):185–9.

49. Jefferson AL, Massaro JM, Wolf PA, et al. Inflammatory biomarkers are associated with total brain volume: the Framingham Heart Study. Neurology 2007 27;68(13):1032–8.

50. Baune BT, Ponath G, Golledge J, et al. Association between IL-8 cytokine and cognitive performance in an elderly general population–the MEMO-Study. Neurobiol Aging 2008;29(6):937–44.

51. Yaffe K, Lindquist K, Penninx BW, et al. Inflammatory markers and cognition in well-functioning African-American and white elders. Neurology 2003;61(1):76–80.

52. Hubbard RE, Woodhouse KW. Frailty, inflammation and the elderly. Biogerontology 2010;11(5):635–41.

53. Leng S, Chaves P, Koenig K, et al. Serum interleukin-6 and hemoglobin as physiological correlates in the geriatric syndrome of frailty: a pilot study. J Am Geriatr Soc 2002;50(7):1268–71.

54. Michaud M, Balardy L, Moulis G, et al. Proinflammatory cytokines, aging, and age-related diseases. J Am Med Dir Assoc 2013;14(12):877–82.

55. Collerton J, Martin-Ruiz C, Davies K, et al. Frailty and the role of inflammation, immunosenescence and cellular ageing in the very old: cross-sectional findings from the Newcastle 85+ Study. Mech Ageing Dev 2012;133(6):456–66.

56. Gómez-Isla T, Hollister R, West H, et al. Neuronal loss correlates with but exceeds neurofibrillary tangles in Alzheimer's disease. Ann Neurol 1997;41(1):17–24.

57. Josephs KA, Whitwell JL, Ahmed Z, et al. Beta-amyloid burden is not associated with rates of brain atrophy. Ann Neurol 2008;63(2):204–12.

58. Mucke L, Selkoe DJ. Neurotoxicity of amyloid β-protein: synaptic and network dysfunction. Cold Spring Harb Perspect Med 2012;2(7):a006338.

59. Laurén J, Gimbel DA, Nygaard HB, et al. Cellular prion protein mediates impairment of synaptic plasticity by amyloid-beta oligomers. Nature 2009;457(7233):1128–32.

60. Shankar GM, Li S, Mehta TH, et al. Amyloid-beta protein dimers isolated directly from Alzheimer's brains impair synaptic plasticity and memory. Nat Med 2008;14(8):837–42.

61. Del Campo N, Payoux P, Djilali A, et al. Relationship of regional brain β-amyloid to gait speed. Neurology 2016;86(1):36–43.

62. Buchman AS, Schneider JA, Leurgans S, et al. Physical frailty in older persons is associated with Alzheimer disease pathology. Neurology 2008;71(7):499–504.
63. Wilson RS, Nag S, Boyle PA, et al. Neural reserve, neuronal density in the locus ceruleus, and cognitive decline. Neurology 2013;80(13):1202–8.
64. Lyness SA, Zarow C, Chui HC. Neuron loss in key cholinergic and aminergic nuclei in Alzheimer disease: a meta-analysis. Neurobiol Aging 2003;24(1):1–23.
65. Buchman AS, Yu L, Wilson RS, et al. Association of brain pathology with the progression of frailty in older adults. Neurology 2013;80(22):2055–61.
66. Mezuk B, Edwards L, Lohman M, et al. Depression and frailty in later life: a synthetic review. Int J Geriatr Psychiatry 2012;27(9):879–92.
67. Paulson D, Lichtenberg PA. Vascular depression: an early warning sign of frailty. Aging Ment Health 2013;17(1):85–93.
68. Lee RSC, Hermens DF, Porter MA, et al. A meta-analysis of cognitive deficits in first-episode Major Depressive Disorder. J Affect Disord 2012;140(2):113–24.
69. Fratiglioni L, Winblad B, von Strauss E. Prevention of Alzheimer's disease and dementia. Major findings from the Kungsholmen Project. Physiol Behav 2007; 92(1–2):98–104.
70. Hertzog C, Kramer A, Wilson R, et al. Enrichment effects on adult cognitive development: can the functional capacity of older adults be preserved and enhanced? Psychol Sci Public Interest 2008;9(1):1–65.
71. Kramer AF, Bherer L, Colcombe SJ, et al. Environmental Influences on cognitive and brain plasticity during aging. J Gerontol A Biol Sci Med Sci 2004;59(9): M940–57.
72. Shulman KI, Herrmann N, Brodaty H, et al. IPA survey of brief cognitive screening instruments. Int Psychogeriatr IPA 2006;18(2):281–94.
73. Folstein MF, Folstein SE, McHugh PR. "Mini-mental state". A practical method for grading the cognitive state of patients for the clinician. J Psychiatr Res 1975; 12(3):189–98.
74. Borson S, Brush M, Gil E, et al. The clock drawing test: utility for dementia detection in multiethnic elders. J Gerontol A Biol Sci Med Sci 1999;54(11):M534–40.
75. Dubois B, Slachevsky A, Litvan I, et al. The FAB: a frontal assessment battery at bedside. Neurology 2000;55(11):1621–6.
76. Dubois B, Touchon J, Portet F, et al. "The 5 words": a simple and sensitive test for the diagnosis of Alzheimer's disease. Presse Med 2002;31(36):1696–9 [in French].
77. Buschke H. Cued recall in amnesia. J Clin Neuropsychol 1984;6(4):433–40.
78. Ricker JH, Axelrod BN. Analysis of an oral paradigm for the trail making test. Assessment 1994;1(1):47–52.
79. Wechsler D. A standardized memory scale for clinical use. J Psychol Interdiscip Appl 1945;19:87–95.
80. Paulsen JS, Butters N, Sadek JR, et al. Distinct cognitive profiles of cortical and subcortical dementia in advanced illness. Neurology 1995;45(5):951–6.
81. Sperling RA, Karlawish J, Johnson KA. Preclinical Alzheimer disease-the challenges ahead. Nat Rev Neurol 2013;9(1):54–8.
82. de Vries NM, Staal JB, van Ravensberg CD, et al. Outcome instruments to measure frailty: a systematic review. Ageing Res Rev 2011;10(1):104–14.
83. Bouillon K, Kivimaki M, Hamer M, et al. Measures of frailty in population-based studies: an overview. BMC Geriatr 2013;13:64.
84. Wilson CJ, Finch CE, Cohen HJ. Cytokines and cognition-the case for a head-to-toe inflammatory paradigm. J Am Geriatr Soc 2002;50(12):2041–56.

85. Engelhart MJ, Geerlings MI, Meijer J, et al. Inflammatory proteins in plasma and the risk of dementia: the rotterdam study. Arch Neurol 2004;61(5):668–72.

86. Ravaglia G, Forti P, Maioli F, et al. Peripheral blood markers of inflammation and functional impairment in elderly community-dwellers. Exp Gerontol 2004;39(9): 1415–22.

87. Desai AK, Grossberg GT, Chibnall JT. Healthy brain aging: a road map. Clin Geriatr Med 2010;26(1):1–16.

88. Landi F, Abbatecola AM, Provinciali M, et al. Moving against frailty: does physical activity matter? Biogerontology 2010;11(5):537–45.

89. Langlois F, Vu TTM, Chassé K, et al. Benefits of physical exercise training on cognition and quality of life in frail older adults. J Gerontol B Psychol Sci Soc Sci 2013;68(3):400–4.

90. Satz P, Morgenstern H, Miller EN, et al. Low education as a possible risk factor for cognitive abnormalities in HIV-1: findings from the multicenter AIDS Cohort Study (MACS). J Acquir Immune Defic Syndr 1993;6(5):503–11.

91. Stern Y. What is cognitive reserve? Theory and research application of the reserve concept. J Int Neuropsychol Soc 2002;8(3):448–60.

92. Stern Y, Albert S, Tang MX, et al. Rate of memory decline in AD is related to education and occupation: cognitive reserve? Neurology 1999;53(9):1942–7.

93. Satz P, Cole MA, Hardy DJ, et al. Brain and cognitive reserve: mediator(s) and construct validity, a critique. J Clin Exp Neuropsychol 2011;33(1):121–30.

94. Hughes CP, Berg L, Danziger WL, et al. A new clinical scale for the staging of dementia. Br J Psychiatry 1982;140:566–72.

95. Morris JC. The clinical dementia rating (CDR): current version and scoring rules. Neurology 1993;43(11):2412–4.

96. Golomb J, Kluger A, Ferris SH. Mild cognitive impairment: historical development and summary of research. Dialogues Clin Neurosci 2004;6(4):351–67.

97. Matthews FE, Stephan BCM, McKeith IG, et al, Medical Research Council Cognitive Function and Ageing Study. Two-year progression from mild cognitive impairment to dementia: to what extent do different definitions agree? J Am Geriatr Soc 2008;56(8):1424–33.

98. Mitchell AJ, Shiri-Feshki M. Rate of progression of mild cognitive impairment to dementia–meta-analysis of 41 robust inception cohort studies. Acta Psychiatr Scand 2009;119(4):252–65.

99. Delrieu J, Andrieu S, Pahor M, et al. Neuropsychological profile of "cognitive frailty" subjects in MAPT study. J Prev Alzheimers Dis 2016;3(3):151–9. Available at: http://www.jpreventionalzheimer.com/all-issues.html?article=192.

100. Canevelli M, Cesari M, van Kan GA. Frailty and cognitive decline: how do they relate? Curr Opin Clin Nutr Metab Care 2015;18(1):43–50.

101. Kamegaya T, Araki Y, Kigure H, et al, Long-Term-Care Prevention Team of Maebashi City. Twelve-week physical and leisure activity programme improved cognitive function in community-dwelling elderly subjects: a randomized controlled trial. Psychogeriatrics 2014;14(1):47–54.

102. Maki Y, Ura C, Yamaguchi T, et al. Effects of intervention using a community-based walking program for prevention of mental decline: a randomized controlled trial. J Am Geriatr Soc 2012;60(3):505–10.

103. Kivipelto M, Solomon A, Ahtiluoto S, et al. The Finnish geriatric intervention study to prevent cognitive impairment and disability (FINGER): study design and progress. Alzheimers Dement 2013;9(6):657–65.

104. Gillette-Guyonnet S, Andrieu S, Dantoine T, et al. Commentary on "A roadmap for the prevention of dementia II. Leon Thal Symposium 2008." the Multidomain

Alzheimer Preventive Trial (MAPT): a new approach to the prevention of Alzheimer's disease. Alzheimers Dement 2009;5(2):114–21.

105. Fitten L. Thinking about cognitive frailty. J Prev Alzheimers Dis 2015;7–10.

106. Alencar MA, Dias JMD, Figueiredo LC, et al. Frailty and cognitive impairment among community-dwelling elderly. Arq Neuropsiquiatr 2013;71(6):362–7.

107. Ferrer A, Badia T, Formiga F, et al. Frailty in the oldest old: prevalence and associated factors. J Am Geriatr Soc 2013;61(2):294–6.

108. Forti P, Maioli F, Lega MV, et al. Combination of the clock drawing test with the physical phenotype of frailty for the prediction of mortality and other adverse outcomes in older community dwellers without dementia. Gerontology 2014; 60(3):204–11.

109. Gray SL, Anderson ML, Hubbard RA, et al. Frailty and incident dementia. J Gerontol A Biol Sci Med Sci 2013;68(9):1083–90.

110. Han ES, Lee Y, Kim J. Association of cognitive impairment with frailty in community-dwelling older adults. Int Psychogeriatr IPA 2014;26(1):155–63.

111. Kulmala J, Nykänen I, Mänty M, et al. Association between frailty and dementia: a population-based study. Gerontology 2014;60(1):16–21.

112. Lee JSW, Auyeung T-W, Leung J, et al. Transitions in frailty states among community-living older adults and their associated factors. J Am Med Dir Assoc 2014;15(4):281–6.

113. McGough EL, Cochrane BB, Pike KC, et al. Dimensions of physical frailty and cognitive function in older adults with amnestic mild cognitive impairment. Ann Phys Rehabil Med 2013;56(5):329–41.

114. Montero-Odasso MM, Barnes B, Speechley M, et al. Disentangling cognitive-frailty: results from the gait and brain study. J Gerontol A Biol Sci Med Sci 2016;71(11):1476–82.

115. Rolfson DB, Wilcock G, Mitnitski A, et al. An assessment of neurocognitive speed in relation to frailty. Age Ageing 2013;42(2):191–6.

116. Runzer-Colmenares FM, Samper-Ternent R, Al Snih S, et al. Prevalence and factors associated with frailty among Peruvian older adults. Arch Gerontol Geriatr 2014;58(1):69–73.

117. Sampson EL, Leurent B, Blanchard MR, et al. Survival of people with dementia after unplanned acute hospital admission: a prospective cohort study. Int J Geriatr Psychiatry 2013;28(10):1015–22.

118. Schoufour JD, van Wijngaarden J, Mitnitski A, et al. Characteristics of the least frail adults with intellectual disabilities: a positive biology perspective. Res Dev Disabil 2014;35(1):127–36.

119. Shimada H, Makizako H, Doi T, et al. Combined prevalence of frailty and mild cognitive impairment in a population of elderly Japanese people. J Am Med Dir Assoc 2013;14(7):518–24.

120. Sourial N, Bergman H, Karunananthan S, et al. Implementing frailty into clinical practice: a cautionary tale. J Gerontol A Biol Sci Med Sci 2013;68(12):1505–11.

Falls in the Aging Population

Kareeann S.F. Khow, MBChB, FRACP, Renuka Visvanathan, MBBS, FRACP, PhD*

KEYWORDS

- Accidental falls • Falls prevention • Older people • Risk factors • Screening

KEY POINTS

- Falls can result in devastating consequences.
- Assessment and remediation of risk factors may prevent falls.
- For those at high risk, comprehensive assessment that includes history of falls; evaluation of medical comorbidities; medication review; physical examination, including gait and balance tests; relevant blood and imaging investigations; and environmental surveillance, is more likely to identify the reasons for falls.
- Multifactorial interventions are more effective than single interventions because the cause of falls is most often a result of multiple interacting factors.

INTRODUCTION

The population is aging globally, and importantly, the rate of increase is greater in developing countries compared with more developed nations.[1] In 2015, about 900 million of the world population was aged 60 years and older, and this is set to increase to more than 2 billion by 2050.[1]

Independence and the ability to "age in place" are fundamentally important for "healthy aging" among older people. Falls and consequential injury or fracture are a threat to "healthy aging," independence, and well-being.

Falls is defined as an event during which a person inadvertently comes to rest on the ground or lower level.[2] Falls are risky to older people, leading to many adverse consequences for the individual. Falls in older people are often a result of interacting risk factors. Falls can be a manifestation of underlying health disorders. Therefore, when older

Disclosure Statement: R. Visvanathan has participated in international initiatives funded by educational grants from Nestle and has presented at symposiums funded by Nestle. She is on the Malnutrition in the Elderly Board with Nestle Australia.

Aged and Extended Care Services, The Queen Elizabeth Hospital, Central Adelaide Local Health Network and Adelaide Geriatrics Training and Research with Aged Care (GTRAC) Centre, School of Medicine, Faculty of Health and Medical Sciences, University of Adelaide, Level 8B, Woodville Road, Woodville South, South Australia 5011, Australia

* Corresponding author.

E-mail address: renuka.visvanathan@adelaide.edu.au

Clin Geriatr Med 33 (2017) 357–368
http://dx.doi.org/10.1016/j.cger.2017.03.002
0749-0690/17/© 2017 Elsevier Inc. All rights reserved.

geriatric.theclinics.com

patients present with falls, it should be seen as an opportunity for a comprehensive assessment to intervene, identify underlying health disorders, and institute strategies to remediate contributory factors.

The impact of falls is not confined to the individual but instead affects families and also the community. The cost of falls on the health care system is phenomenal, and therefore, it is not surprising that falls prevention and management strategies are considered vital for many health and aged care systems internationally.

Reassuringly, there is growing evidence to support falls prevention and management activities, but the challenge remains with the translation of evidence. A failure to act at this time will contribute to increasing disability, mortality, and costs for the aging population. In contrast, effective translation of available evidence might prevent falls and its consequences, which in turn will enable the achievement of "healthy aging."

This review, which focuses on assessing risk of falls in community-dwelling older people, seeks to highlight the impact of falls, discusses some of the risk factors, and finally, concludes by providing an overview of intervention strategies.

PREVALENCE, LOCATION, AND CONSEQUENCES

It is estimated that a third of community-dwelling individuals older than 65 years fall each year, and this increases to a reported rate of 50% in some studies of those living in residential care facilities.[3] About 40% of people aged 80 years and over may suffer from at least one fall each year.[4] In hospital, fall rates vary between 3 and 20 per 1000 bed-days.[5] Therefore, falls are common.

Most falls occur during the day and at home, with 20% occurring at night between 9 PM and 7 AM, some involving a rush to the bathroom.[6] Another study identified transitions between surfaces (eg, on, to, or from carpet/rug or wet areas)[7] and entry into and out of motor vehicles as other risk locations.[8] Getting on and off furniture can also be risky (eg, chairs or stools or bed).[8]

Falls are the main contributor to injury, related disability, and premature death in older people.[4] Severity of injuries can vary, and 40% to 60% of falls result in major lacerations, nonvertebral fractures, and traumatic head injuries.[9] Prolonged lying after a fall can lead to dehydration, rhabdomyolysis, pressure sores, and pneumonia, all of which add to the length of hospital stay.[10] There is also an association between falls and the sequential occurrence of radial, humeral, or vertebral fractures and hip fractures (ie, the "fracture cascade").[11] Almost 95% of all hip fractures are a result of falls.[12] An estimated 10% to 20% of patients with hip fractures are discharged to nursing homes, and 20% die within 12 months.[13,14]

Falls not only result in physical injury but also cause psychological injury whereby falls lead to a "fear" of falling.[15] This "fear" can develop in 20% to 40% of people who fall, cause debility, and lead to a downward spiral of physical health, resulting in functional decline, social isolation, depression, and institutionalization.[15]

The human and economic costs of falls are well reported globally. In the United States, falls are the second leading cause of unintentional death (after road traffic injuries) from injury and the leading cause of nonfatal injury.[16] In the United Kingdom, falls account for about 14% of emergency admissions, 4% of all hospital admissions in people more than 65 years, and approximately one-third of all injury-related hospitalizations.[17] In Australia, within the Sydney metropolitan area, 37,488 fall-related ambulance calls were recorded in a 2008 public health surveillance database, translating to a crude rate of 843 per 100,000 people.[18] Fifty-six percent of these calls were deemed priority code 1, thus requiring an immediate response. In 2013, the US Centers for Disease Control and Prevention (CDC) reported that there were 2.5 million nonfatal falls among older people presenting to the emergency departments, 734,000 hospitalizations, and a direct medical cost of $30 billion.[16] These estimated costs increase substantially when indirect costs such as lost productivity and costs borne by the patient, family, and community are included.

RISK FACTORS FOR FALLS

The risk of falling increases with the number of risk factors present in each individual.[19] From a clinical perspective, the comprehensive clinical assessment is assisted by the systematic classification of risk factors for falls as intrinsic (individual-related) and extrinsic (external to the individual) factors (**Table 1**). Here, the authors focus on some intrinsic factors.

Sensory Impairment

Visual impairment, especially impaired depth perception and loss of contrast sensitivity, has been identified as one of the strongest risk factors for multiple falls in community-dwelling older adults.[20] Evidence has shown that expedited cataract surgery in the first eye and switching from bifocal or multifocal to single-lens glasses reduced the rates of falls.[21,22]

Hearing loss is also associated with significantly increased odds of falling in older adults.[23] This association can be explained by an underlying vestibular abnormality, impaired balance given the reduced cognitive load of hearing loss, and a loss of auditory perception leading to reduced spatial awareness.[23]

Epidemiologic data demonstrate that dual sensory impairment (visual and hearing) significantly increases the risk of falls.[24] Sadly, many older people fail to gain timely access to optometrist, audiology, and ophthalmology services. Redesign of health care services should occur to improve timely access.

Table 1
Risk factors for falls in older people

Intrinsic Factors	Extrinsic Factors
Demographics	Personal care
Advanced age	Polypharmacy
Female	Inappropriate footwear
Physical health	Bifocals or multifocals
Gait and balance impairment	Environment
Slow gait speed	Inappropriate walking aids
Sarcopenia	Home hazards
Frailty	Outdoor hazards
Psychological health	Social
Cognitive impairment	Lives alone
Depression	Sedentary behavior
Fear of falling	Poor support network
Sensory impairment	
Visual impairment	
Hearing impairment	
Comorbid illnesses (common examples)	
Neurologic disorders	
Arthropathy	
Anemia	
Diabetes mellitus	

Sedentary Behavior

Sedentary behavior occurs when a person's activity does not result in a substantial increase in energy expenditure above resting level (<1.5 metabolic equivalent of task).[25] These activities occur predominantly in a sitting or reclined position (ie, television viewing, reading). Studies have shown that older people are sedentary more than 70% of the time, that is, 8 to 10 hours of the waking day, and that sedentary behavior increases with age.[26] Higher level of sedentary duration, particularly if more than 10 h/ d, is associated with increased risk of falls in older people with mobility limitation.[27] This observation was also supported by a meta-analysis.[28] Measures are required to encourage exercise and physical activity as part of health promotion.

Frailty, Nutrition, and Oral Health

In older age, there is a reduction in appetite (ie, from anorexia of aging) and nutrient (including protein) intake leading to not only a loss of muscle mass but also performance (ie, sarcopenia).[29] Sarcopenia is an independent risk factor for falls in older adults living in the community.[30] Poor oral health is also associated with poor nutritional status and sarcopenia.[31] Reduced muscle strength and mass are features associated with phenotypic frailty. There is a bidirectional association between frailty and falls.[32] Frailty is characterized by diminished strength, diminished endurance, and reduced physiologic function that increases an individual's vulnerability for developing increased dependency or death.[33] Frail older adults may fall because of balance impairment or reduced muscle strength.[32]

Cognition and Mood Disorders

A meta-analysis indicates that cognitive impairment is associated with higher risk of falls.[34] The risk of falling increases by 20% for every reduction of point in the Mini Mental State Examination.[35] Executive dysfunction, impairment in dual tasking, information processing, and reaction time are associated with increased risk of falling.[36] Depression is also associated with increased falls risk.[37] Older adults suffering from depression, either due to or as a result of other medical conditions such as stroke, Parkinson disease, or dementia, are at increased risk of falls. A pilot study has shown that patients with depression have slower gait speed, reduced ability to dual task, and impaired executive function, which are associated with higher risk of falls.[38]

Gait, Balance, and Neurologic Impairment

Disorders of gait and balance are consistently strong predictors for falls.[39] As part of aging, the gait pattern becomes more rigid and less coordinated with reduced posture control.[40] Muscle strength, step length, and reflexes are also reduced.[41,42] Older patients with neurologic disorders affecting their gait are at increased risk of falls (eg, parkinsonian, peripheral neuropathy, foot drop, hemiparesis, frontal lobe disorders, and spasticity).[43] Peripheral neuropathy might occur as a result of treatable conditions, such as diabetes mellitus, vitamin B_{12} deficiency, and hypothyroidism, and increase the risk of falling.

Vitamin D insufficiency is highly prevalent especially in the older population at higher risk of falls. It is postulated that vitamin D insufficiency is associated with reductions not only in both bone mineral density (BMD) but also in reduced muscle strength, leading to increased risk of falls and fractures.[44] Therefore, vitamin D replacement is beneficial in older people who are deficient in this vitamin. However, the efficacy of vitamin D supplementation in reducing falls risk is controversial due to the heterogeneity of vitamin D dose in trials and variable repletion dose among individuals.[45,46] Vitamin

D supplementation with 800 IU in combination with a calcium-rich diet can be recommended in all older adults to optimize bone health.

Comorbid Illness

Orthostatic hypotension (OSH) is an important risk factor for falls because it affects up to 30% of the population over the age of 65 years.[47] It is defined as a drop in systolic blood pressure (SBP) of at least 20 mm Hg or diastolic blood pressure of 10 mm Hg within 3 minutes of standing.[47] One study reported that older people with systolic OSH at 1 minute were at greater risk of falls.[48] Another risk factor for falls frequently not recognized is postprandial hypotension.[49] It is defined as a 20-mm Hg reduction in SBP or a decline in SBP to less than 90 mm Hg from a preingestion SBP of greater than 100 mm Hg, occurring within 120 minutes of meal commencement.[49]

Falls can also be related to rhythm disorders, such as atrioventricular block, carotid sinus hypersensitivity, and sick sinus syndrome.[50,51] Several studies have also found an association between anemia and increased risk of falls and falls-related injuries.[52,53]

SCREENING AND ASSESSMENT OF FALLS

The American and British Geriatrics Societies and the Australian Commission on Safety and Quality in Health Care have published clinical practice guidelines on fall risk screening and assessment.[54,55] For community-dwelling older people, most guidelines recommend annual screening initiated by primary care or health care providers in all people aged 65 and above. The rationale behind this is that early identification of risk allows for earlier institution of strategies to mitigate that risk.

The CDC has developed a "Stay Independent Brochure," which includes a modified falls risk questionnaire consisting of 12 questions that the older person can complete.[56] Those scoring 4 or more in the questionnaire are considered to have screened positive for falls risk and are encouraged to discuss the questionnaire with their general practitioner (GP). Once they approach their GP, the STEADI (Stopping Elderly Accidents, Deaths, and Injuries) algorithm is applied.[56] Those answering yes to any of the key questions highlighted in **Box 1** will need to at least undergo the Timed Up and Go Test (TUGT) to evaluate for gait, strength, and balance.[57] A self-reported Fall Risk Questionnaire is another useful tool in the initial assessment of people at risk of falls.[58]

Low Risk

Patients presenting to their GP with a normal TUGT (ie, <12 seconds) but with either "no" or some "yes" responses to key questions should receive education, vitamin D, and/or calcium where there is a need and be encouraged to participate in strength and balance exercise classes.

Box 1
Screening questions for risk of falls

1. Any falls in the past year? If YES, ask:
   a. How many times?
   b. Were you injured?

2. Any unsteadiness when walking or standing?

3. Any worries about falling?

From US Centers for Disease Control and Prevention (CDC) Stopping Elderly Accidents, Deaths and Injuries (STEADI) algorithm and Stevens JA, Phelan EA. Development of STEADI: a fall prevention resource for health care providers. Health Promot Pract 2013;14:706–14.

High Risk

Those with an abnormal TUGT and 2 or more falls or one injurious fall in the last year will undergo a comprehensive assessment with a care plan developed. A comprehensive falls risk assessment consists of a detailed falls history, general and fall-focused physical examination, medication review, nutritional assessment, frailty, functional assessment, home and environmental assessments, relevant investigations, and bone health assessment. Multiple screening tools can be used to identify risk, and where risk is identified, a more detailed assessment of that condition will be necessary to guide treatment. These high-risk individuals should be reviewed within 30 days to monitor for change and update the care plan.

Falls history

A falls history should include frequency of falls in the past year, circumstances around the fall or falls (eg, time, location, activity when fall or falls occurred, preceding symptoms, type of footwear) and consequences of falls (eg, injuries, fear of falling, pain or activity restriction). Corroborative history from caregivers or family members can be useful in the assessment of recurrent and unexplained falls.

Functional and continence assessment

The TUGT is an ideal test because it allows for observation of the older person's ability to get off a chair and sit back in it. It also allows for an observation of balance and gait. Slowing of gait can also be monitored for. In addition, an assessment of activities of daily living should be made using validated scales, such as the Lawton and Katz scales.[59,60] The physical activity scale for the elderly or a pedometer is also useful to encourage increased participation in physical activity or exercise.[61] Urinary incontinence should be assessed and treated where relevant.

Nutrition, appetite, and sarcopenia assessment

The Mini Nutritional Assessment has been validated for use in older people, and a short form that provides an alternate for calf circumference measurement instead of body mass index exists and should be used to screen for undernutrition.[62] To detect impairment of appetite that might predate weight loss, the Simplified Nutritional Appetite Questionnaire is a validated tool that consists of 4 simple questions (appetite, fullness, taste, and number of meals), which takes less than 2 minutes to complete.[63] The SARC-F (Strength, Assistance with walking, Rise from a chair, Ambulation, Climb stairs and Falls) is a simple questionnaire that is easily administered and able to detect those at-risk of sarcopenia (ie, score $\geq$4).[64]

Cognition and mood

A brief cognitive screen such as the rapid cognitive screen, abbreviated mental test, or Mini-Cog can be used to screen for cognitive impairment.[65–67] The 5-item geriatric depression scale can be used to screen for depression risk.[68] Improving one's mood will be important if a person is to participate in and adhere to treatment strategies. The Hospital and Anxiety Depression Scale anxiety subscale might be useful in screening for anxiety.[69]

Fracture risk assessment

Older people at high risk of falls should be assessed for future fracture risk and evaluated for osteoporosis. The World Health Organization has produced the FRAX (Fracture Risk Assessment Tool) calculator as a tool to assess people who are at risk of fragility fractures.[70] Individuals with probabilities for major osteoporotic fracture and/or hip fracture at or above the intervention threshold should be treated according to country-specific thresholds.[70] It has been suggested that the FRAX alone provides the same prediction of future osteoporotic fracture probability as FRAX in combination with BMD assessment.[71] However, FRAX may underestimate fracture risk because it does not incorporate falls history or number of previous fractures. Alternative calculators like the Garvan Bone Fracture Risk Calculator derived from the Dubbo Osteoporosis Epidemiology Study may be more useful in people with multiple falls.[72] BMD assessment using dual-energy x-ray absorptiometry (DXA) is useful for those at intermediate risk whereby DXA may help the clinician reach a decision to treat or not treat.

Medications review

The number, type, dose, and mode of administration of all medications, including over-the-counter medications, should be reviewed. The use of tools such as the STOPP (Screening Tool of Older Person's Prescription)/START (Screening Tool to Alert Doctors to Right Treatment) criteria to guide appropriate prescribing should be considered.[73] Special attention should be given to avoid psychoactive medications because these agents can be sedating, alter sensorium, and impair balance and gait.[74] Optimal blood pressure management is ideal, but hypotension should be avoided. Similarly, pain should be well managed to encourage exercise, but on the other hand, side effects such as sedation and hypotension should be cautioned.

Frailty

Frailty risk can be assessed using the FRAIL (Fatigue, Resistance, Ambulation, Incontinence, Loss of weight) screen that is a simple questionnaire that can be completed quickly and the questions mirror those assessed through the phenotypic method.[75] With the aid of information technology, the comprehensive assessments suggested above when completed electronically could be used to generate a frailty index score, which can be used to monitor for change in frailty risk over time.[76]

Comprehensive physical examination

Box 2 summarizes the important aspects of performing a comprehensive physical examination of falls risk. Each eye should be tested independently and with glasses if present. Near vision can be tested by holding a Rosenbaum card at 36 cm, and distance vision can be tested by using a Snellen chart at 6 m. An electrocardiography should be performed in those with cardiovascular diseases or at high risk of cardiac arrhythmias. A urinalysis could be undertaken to rule out infection.

Box 2
Essential aspects of a fall-focused physical examination

- Orthostatic and postprandial blood pressure
- Visual acuity, field, and oculomotor movements
- Auditory assessment
- Cardiac examination (rate, rhythm, murmurs)
- Musculoskeletal examination of back and lower extremities
  - Range of movement
- Neurologic examination
  - Muscle bulk, tone, power, reflexes
  - Coordination
  - Sensation: Pinprick, light touch, and proprioception
  - Balance, including Romberg's
- Cognition assessment

Home and environmental assessment

Home and environmental assessment is an essential component of falls assessment and helps identify extrinsic risk factors for falls.[77] Risks such as poor lighting, slippery surfaces, clutter, and rugs might be identified. The need for seat raises, ramps, and railings might also be identified. In a meta-analysis, providing home environmental intervention was shown to reduce the risk of falls by 21%, and the reduction was greater in those at high risk of falling.[78]

Laboratory and imaging investigations

There might be a need for routine laboratory testing to ascertain any anemia, hyponatremia, hypovitaminosis (vitamin D and B_{12}), hypoglycemia, hypothyroidism, and renal failure. Computed tomography or MRI of the brain is indicated if there is evidence of neurologic deficit or if dementia is suspected.

INTERVENTIONS FOR FALLS PREVENTION

The objectives of managing falls risk are to reduce falls, reduce the risk of injury, and maintain the highest possible level of independence. Multifactorial interventions may involve a combination of exercise programs, balance training, medications review, home risk modifications, and education. The right footwear as well as orthoses is important.[79] One systematic review found that older adults who wore slippers had a higher falls risk than those who walked barefoot or with fastened shoes.[80] In one systematic review of 19 trials involving multifactorial interventions for falls risk, a 14% reduction in the rate of falls was noted.[77] As already discussed, it is likely that the approach taken should be individualized after a holistic assessment. Implementation of falls prevention strategies requires a team effort involving a multidisciplinary team. Exercise programs that focus on strength training and balance have been shown in a meta-analysis to be most effective in reducing falls rate and should be encouraged as a falls prevention strategy.[81] Other exercise programs such as Tai Chi can also reduce risk of falls by targeting the balance, but no long-term data are available yet.[82] However, one of the greatest challenges is in encouraging ongoing adherence to an exercise program. Technology-based intervention and monitoring are increasingly being integrated into falls prevention programs and may be beneficial. There is a need for health professionals to develop the knowledge, skills, and competency to recognize falls risk and prevent falls. It therefore follows that undergraduate and continued professional development curriculum should include core content in relation to falls risk recognition and management.

SUMMARY

Falls in older people are common and usually multifactorial in cause. Falls are a complex and costly public health issue. Screening in the community is beneficial for early identification. For older people at risk of falls, a comprehensive approach in assessment is often required followed by a multidisciplinary and multidomain intervention.

ACKNOWLEDGMENTS

The authors thank Dr Pazhvoor Shibu for reviewing and providing feedback on the article.

REFERENCES

1. United Nations, Department of Economics and Social Affairs. World population ageing 2015. New York: United Nations; 2015.

2. World Health Organization. WHO global report on falls prevention in older age. Geneva: World Health Organization; 2007.
3. Tromp AM, Pluijm SM, Smit JH, et al. Fall-risk screening test: a prospective study on predictors for falls in community-dwelling elderly. J Clin Epidemiol 2001;54:837–44.
4. Tinetti ME, Williams CS. The effect of falls and fall injuries on functioning in community-dwelling older persons. J Gerontol A Biol Sci Med Sci 1998;53: M112–9.
5. Vassallo M, Azeem T, Pirwani MF, et al. An epidemiological study of falls on integrated general medical wards. Int J Clin Pract 2000;54:654–7.
6. Campbell AJ, Borrie MJ, Spears GF, et al. Circumstances and consequences of falls experienced by a community population 70 years and over during a prospective study. Age Ageing 1990;19:136–41.
7. Rosen T, Mack KA, Noonan RK. Slipping and tripping: fall injuries in adults associated with rugs and carpets. J Inj Violence Res 2013;5(1):61–9.
8. Dellinger AM, Boyd RM, Haileyesus T. Fall injuries in older adults from an unusual source: entering and exiting a vehicle. J Am Geriatr Soc 2008;56:609–14.
9. Masud T, Morris RO. Epidemiology of falls. Age Ageing 2001;30(Suppl 4):3–7.
10. Fleming J, Brayne C. Inability to get up after falling, subsequent time on floor, and summoning help: prospective cohort study in people over 90. BMJ 2008;337: a2227.
11. Melton LJ 3rd, Amin S. Is there a specific fracture 'cascade'? Bonekey Rep 2013; 2:367.
12. Cummings SR, Melton LJ. Epidemiology and outcomes of osteoporotic fractures. Lancet 2002;359:1761–7.
13. Sattui SE, Saag KG. Fracture mortality: associations with epidemiology and osteoporosis treatment. Nat Rev Endocrinol 2014;10:592–602.
14. Vochteloo AJ, van Vliet-Koppert ST, Maier AB, et al. Risk factors for failure to return to the pre-fracture place of residence after hip fracture: a prospective longitudinal study of 444 patients. Arch Orthop Trauma Surg 2012;132:823–30.
15. Scheffer AC, Schuurmans MJ, van Dijk N, et al. Fear of falling: measurement strategy, prevalence, risk factors and consequences among older persons. Age Ageing 2008;37:19–24.
16. Center for Disease Control and Prevention. Cost of falls among older adults. Available at: http://www.cdc.gov/homeandrecreationalsafety/falls/fallcost.html. Accessed August 30, 2016.
17. Close J, Ellis M, Hooper R, et al. Prevention of falls in the elderly trial (PROFET): a randomised controlled trial. Lancet 1999;353:93–7.
18. Thomas SL, Muscatello DJ, Middleton PM, et al. Characteristics of fall-related injuries attended by an ambulance in Sydney, Australia: a surveillance summary. N S W Public Health Bull 2011;22:49–54.
19. Ambrose AF, Paul G, Hausdorff JM. Risk factors for falls among older adults: a review of the literature. Maturitas 2013;75:51–61.
20. Salonen L, Kivela SL. Eye diseases and impaired vision as possible risk factors for recurrent falls in the aged: a systematic review. Curr Gerontol Geriatr Res 2012;2012:271481.
21. Harwood RH, Foss AJ, Osborn F, et al. Falls and health status in elderly women following first eye cataract surgery: a randomised controlled trial. Br J Ophthalmol 2005;89:53–9.
22. Lord SR, Dayhew J, Howland A. Multifocal glasses impair edge-contrast sensitivity and depth perception and increase the risk of falls in older people. J Am Geriatr Soc 2002;50:1760–6.

23. Jiam NT, Li C, Agrawal Y. Hearing loss and falls: a systematic review and meta-analysis. Laryngoscope 2016;126(11):2587–96.
24. Gopinath B, McMahon CM, Burlutsky G, et al. Hearing and vision impairment and the 5-year incidence of falls in older adults. Age Ageing 2016;45:409–14.
25. Pate RR, O'Neill JR, Lobelo F. The evolving definition of "sedentary". Exerc Sport Sci Rev 2008;36:173–8.
26. van der Ploeg HP, Chey T, Korda RJ, et al. Sitting time and all-cause mortality risk in 222 497 Australian adults. Arch Intern Med 2012;172:494–500.
27. Cauley JA, Harrison SL, Cawthon PM, et al. Objective measures of physical activity, fractures and falls: the osteoporotic fractures in men study. J Am Geriatr Soc 2013;61:1080–8.
28. Thibaud M, Bloch F, Tournoux-Facon C, et al. Impact of physical activity and sedentary behaviour on fall risks in older people: a systematic review and meta-analysis of observational studies. Eur Rev Aging Phys Act 2012;9:5–15.
29. Visvanathan R, Chapman I. Preventing sarcopaenia in older people. Maturitas 2010;66:383–8.
30. Landi F, Liperoti R, Russo A, et al. Sarcopenia as a risk factor for falls in elderly individuals: results from the ilSIRENTE study. Clin Nutr 2012;31:652–8.
31. Poisson P, Laffond T, Campos S, et al. Relationships between oral health, dysphagia and undernutrition in hospitalised elderly patients. Gerodontology 2016;33:161–8.
32. Kojima G. Frailty as a predictor of future falls among community-dwelling older people: a systematic review and meta-analysis. J Am Med Dir Assoc 2015;16:1027–33.
33. Clegg A, Young J, Iliffe S, et al. Frailty in elderly people. Lancet 2013;381:752–62.
34. Muir SW, Gopaul K, Montero Odasso MM. The role of cognitive impairment in fall risk among older adults: a systematic review and meta-analysis. Age Ageing 2012;41:299–308.
35. Gleason CE, Gangnon RE, Fischer BL, et al. Increased risk for falling associated with subtle cognitive impairment: secondary analysis of a randomized clinical trial. Dement Geriatr Cogn Disord 2009;27:557–63.
36. Mirelman A, Herman T, Brozgol M, et al. Executive function and falls in older adults: new findings from a five-year prospective study link fall risk to cognition. PLoS One 2012;7:e40297.
37. Stubbs B, Stubbs J, Gnanaraj SD, et al. Falls in older adults with major depressive disorder (MDD): a systematic review and exploratory meta-analysis of prospective studies. Int Psychogeriatr 2016;28:23–9.
38. Paleacu D, Shutzman A, Giladi N, et al. Effects of pharmacological therapy on gait and cognitive function in depressed patients. Clin Neuropharmacol 2007;30:63–71.
39. Deandrea S, Lucenteforte E, Bravi F, et al. Risk factors for falls in community-dwelling older people: a systematic review and meta-analysis. Epidemiology 2010;21:658–68.
40. Barak Y, Wagenaar RC, Holt KG. Gait characteristics of elderly people with a history of falls: a dynamic approach. Phys Ther 2006;86:1501–10.
41. Jensen JL, Brown LA, Woollacott MH. Compensatory stepping: the biomechanics of a preferred response among older adults. Exp Aging Res 2001;27:361–76.
42. Verghese J, Holtzer R, Lipton RB, et al. Quantitative gait markers and incident fall risk in older adults. J Gerontol A Biol Sci Med Sci 2009;64:896–901.
43. Verghese J, Ambrose AF, Lipton RB, et al. Neurological gait abnormalities and risk of falls in older adults. J Neurol 2010;257:392–8.
44. Sanders KM, Scott D, Ebeling PR. Vitamin D deficiency and its role in muscle-bone interactions in the elderly. Curr Osteoporos Rep 2014;12:74–81.

45. Bischoff-Ferrari HA, Dawson-Hughes B, Staehelin HB, et al. Fall prevention with supplemental and active forms of vitamin D: a meta-analysis of randomised controlled trials. BMJ 2009;339:b3692.

46. Latham NK, Anderson CS, Reid IR. Effects of vitamin D supplementation on strength, physical performance, and falls in older persons: a systematic review. J Am Geriatr Soc 2003;51:1219–26.

47. Mukai S, Lipsitz LA. Orthostatic hypotension. Clin Geriatr Med 2002;18:253–68.

48. Gangavati A, Hajjar I, Quach L, et al. Hypertension, orthostatic hypotension, and the risk of falls in a community-dwelling elderly population: the maintenance of balance, independent living, intellect, and zest in the elderly of Boston study. J Am Geriatr Soc 2011;59(3):383–9.

49. Trahair LG, Horowitz M, Jones KL. Postprandial hypotension: a systematic review. J Am Med Dir Assoc 2014;15:394–409.

50. Kenny RA, Richardson DA. Carotid sinus syndrome and falls in older adults. Am J Geriatr Cardiol 2001;10:97–9.

51. Seifer C, Kenny RA. The prevalence of falls in older persons paced for atrioventricular block and sick sinus syndrome. Am J Geriatr Cardiol 2003;12:298–301.

52. Bowling CB, Muntner P, Bradbury BD, et al. Low hemoglobin levels and recurrent falls in U.S. men and women: prospective findings from the REasons for Geographic and Racial Differences in Stroke (REGARDS) cohort. Am J Med Sci 2013;345:446–54.

53. Duh MS, Mody SH, Lefebvre P, et al. Anaemia and the risk of injurious falls in a community-dwelling elderly population. Drugs Aging 2008;25:325–34.

54. Bjorkelund KB, Hommel A, Thorngren KG, et al. The influence of perioperative care and treatment on the 4-month outcome in elderly patients with hip fracture. AANA J 2011;79:51–61.

55. Australian Commission on Safety and Quality in Health Care. Safety and quality improvement guide standard 10: preventing falls and harm from falls (October 2012). Sydney (Australia): ACSQHC; 2012.

56. Stevens JA, Phelan EA. Development of STEADI: a fall prevention resource for health care providers. Health Promot Pract 2013;14:706–14.

57. Shumway-Cook A, Brauer S, Woollacott M. Predicting the probability for falls in community-dwelling older adults using the Timed up & Go Test. Phys Ther 2000;80:896–903.

58. Rubenstein LZ, Vivrette R, Harker JO, et al. Validating an evidence-based, self-rated fall risk questionnaire (FRQ) for older adults. J Safety Res 2011;42:493–9.

59. Katz S, Ford AB, Moskowitz RW, et al. Studies of illness in the aged. The index of ADL: a standardized measure of biological and psychological function. JAMA 1963;185:914–9.

60. Lawton MP, Brody EM. Assessment of older people: self-maintaining and instrumental activities of daily living. Gerontologist 1969;9:179–86.

61. Washburn RA, McAuley E, Katula J, et al. The physical activity scale for the elderly (PASE): evidence for validity. J Clin Epidemiol 1999;52:643–51.

62. Dent E, Visvanathan R, Piantadosi C, et al. Nutritional screening tools as predictors of mortality, functional decline, and move to higher level care in older people: a systematic review. J Nutr Gerontol Geriatr 2012;31:97–145.

63. Kruizenga HM, Seidell JC, de Vet HC, et al. Development and validation of a hospital screening tool for malnutrition: the short nutritional assessment questionnaire (SNAQ). Clin Nutr 2005;24:75–82.

64. Malmstrom TK, Miller DK, Simonsick EM, et al. SARC-F: a symptom score to predict persons with sarcopenia at risk for poor functional outcomes. J Cachexia Sarcopenia Muscle 2016;7:28–36.
65. Hodkinson HM. Evaluation of a mental test score for assessment of mental impairment in the elderly. Age Ageing 1972;1:233–8.
66. Borson S, Scanlan JM, Chen P, et al. The Mini-Cog as a screen for dementia: validation in a population-based sample. J Am Geriatr Soc 2003;51:1451–4.
67. Malmstrom TK, Voss VB, Cruz-Oliver DM, et al. The rapid cognitive screen (RCS): a point-of-care screening for dementia and mild cognitive impairment. J Nutr Health Aging 2015;19:741–4.
68. Song HJ, Meade K, Akobundu U, et al. Depression as a correlate of functional status of community-dwelling older adults: utilizing a short-version of 5-item Geriatric Depression Scale as a screening tool. J Nutr Health Aging 2014;18:765–70.
69. Wetherell JL, Birchler GD, Ramsdell J, et al. Screening for generalized anxiety disorder in geriatric primary care patients. Int J Geriatr Psychiatry 2007;22:115–23.
70. Kanis JA, Harvey NC, Cooper C, et al. A systematic review of intervention thresholds based on FRAX: a report prepared for the National Osteoporosis Guideline Group and the International Osteoporosis Foundation. Arch Osteoporos 2016;11:25.
71. Gadam RK, Schlauch K, Izuora KE. Frax prediction without BMD for assessment of osteoporotic fracture risk. Endocr Pract 2013;19(5):780–4.
72. Nguyen ND, Frost SA, Center JR, et al. Development of prognostic nomograms for individualizing 5-year and 10-year fracture risks. Osteoporos Int 2008;19:1431–44.
73. O'Mahony D, O'Sullivan D, Byrne S, et al. STOPP/START criteria for potentially inappropriate prescribing in older people: version 2. Age Ageing 2015;44:213–8.
74. Glab KL, Wooding FG, Tuiskula KA. Medication-related falls in the elderly: mechanisms and prevention strategies. Consult Pharm 2014;29:413–7.
75. Woo J, Yu R, Wong M, et al. Frailty screening in the community using the FRAIL scale. J Am Med Dir Assoc 2015;16:412–9.
76. Jones DM, Song X, Rockwood K. Operationalizing a frailty index from a standardized comprehensive geriatric assessment. J Am Geriatr Soc 2004;52:1929–33.
77. Gillespie LD, Robertson MC, Gillespie WJ, et al. Interventions for preventing falls in older people living in the community. Cochrane Database Syst Rev 2012;(9):CD007146.
78. Clemson L, Mackenzie L, Ballinger C, et al. Environmental interventions to prevent falls in community-dwelling older people: a meta-analysis of randomized trials. J Aging Health 2008;20:954–71.
79. Cakar E, Durmus O, Tekin L, et al. The ankle-foot orthosis improves balance and reduces fall risk of chronic spastic hemiparetic patients. Eur J Phys Rehabil Med 2010;46:363–8.
80. Menant JC, Steele JR, Menz HB, et al. Optimizing footwear for older people at risk of falls. J Rehabil Res Dev 2008;45:1167–81.
81. El-Khoury F, Cassou B, Charles MA, et al. The effect of fall prevention exercise programmes on fall induced injuries in community dwelling older adults: systematic review and meta-analysis of randomised controlled trials. BMJ 2013;347:f6234.
82. Voukelatos A, Cumming RG, Lord SR, et al. A randomized, controlled trial of tai chi for the prevention of falls: the Central Sydney tai chi trial. J Am Geriatr Soc 2007;55:1185–91.

Rapid Geriatric Assessment of Hip Fracture

Jesse Zanker, MBBS, BMedSci[a], Gustavo Duque, MD, PhD[a,b,c],*

KEYWORDS

- Hip fracture • Osteoporosis • Elderly • Orthogeriatrics • Assessment
- Preoperative assessment • Morbidity • Mortality

KEY POINTS

- A comprehensive multidimensional preoperative assessment should be performed in all hip fracture patients.
- Use of risk predictors is highly recommended in order to identify potential postoperative complications.
- Long-term complications could be also predicted and prevented by a comprehensive preoperative assessment.

PREOPERATIVE ASSESSMENT

Hip fracture should be suspected in any older person experiencing hip, groin, or femur pain and inability to mobilize following a fall or trauma.[1] The preoperative assessment should focus on rapidly gathering information to promptly optimize the patient for surgery. The role of the geriatrician is to thoroughly evaluate the patient for acute and chronic illness[2] and address medical issues that will impact upon intraoperative and postoperative morbidity and mortality. The geriatrician may form an integral part of the multidisciplinary care pathway, which is a complex intervention that can optimize clinical outcomes and resource use.[3–5] In patients with hip fracture, care pathways reduce in-hospital mortality, medical complications, wound infections, and pressure sores.[6]

Disclosure: Prof. G. Duque is a consultant for Amgen, Sanofi, and Lilly Australia.
[a] Department of Aged Care, Sunshine Hospital, Western Health, 176 Furlong Road, St. Albans, Victoria 3021, Australia; [b] Australian Institute for Musculoskeletal Science (AIMSS), Level 3, Centre for Health, Research and Education, Sunshine Hospital, Western Health, The University of Melbourne, 176 Furlong Road, St. Albans, Victoria 3021, Australia; [c] Department of Medicine-Western Precinct, Melbourne Medical School, The University of Melbourne, 176 Furlong Road, St Albans, Victoria 3021, Australia
* Corresponding author. Department of Aged Care, Sunshine Hospital, Western Health, 176 Furlong Road, St. Albans, Victoria 3021, Australia.
E-mail address: gustavo.duque@unimelb.edu.au

Timing of Surgery

Studies examining time to surgery and outcomes following hip fracture have been observational in nature and results have been conflicting.[7–15] However, 3 systematic reviews have found that operative delay (beyond 48 hours in 2 reviews) significantly increased in-hospital and 1-year mortality.[16–18] Early surgery improved length of stay, reduced pressure sores, and increased the likelihood of a return to independent living.[7,17,18] The exception to early surgery is in patients with active high-risk cardiac conditions (**Box 1**), who should undergo additional preoperative assessment and possible delay to surgery to achieve optimization in order to improve outcomes.[19] However, the benefits of any intervention that delays surgery should be balanced with the knowledge that surgical delay generally results in poorer outcomes.[20]

Components of the Preoperative Assessment

History

Establishing a comprehensive understanding of the medical, social, and functional history in addition to the circumstances of the mechanism of injury is integral to the preoperative assessment. Preoperative delirium and preexisting dementia are obstacles to accurate history taking and may be present in more than 50% and 30% of patients with hip fracture, respectively.[21] Collateral history from important others or witnesses will often be required. Retrieving relevant information from the family physician and involved specialists should also form part of the history-taking process.

The medical history should also focus on active conditions or those that may reemerge intraoperatively or postoperatively, along with review of body systems and medications. A focused falls history should include inquiring about prodromal symptoms, active illness, environmental factors, contributory chronic conditions, and medications known to increase risk of falls.[22] Additional risks, such as urinary incontinence, visual impairment, footwear, and alcohol intake, should be explored.[22]

Establishing the patient's prehospital basic and instrumental activities of daily living (ADLs) guides the development of goals designed to achieve premorbid function in postoperative rehabilitation and may provide a surrogate predictor of mortality risk.[23] Following hip fracture, there is a reduction in the ability to undertake ADLs of approximately 15% to 20% in surviving patients at 1 year following fracture.[23] Mortality is highest among those with lower functional performance.[23]

Cognition

Patients with preexisting dementia are more likely to experience delirium in the perioperative phase.[24] Delirium increases the risk of death, institutionalization, and

---

Box 1
High-risk cardiac conditions requiring further evaluation and treatment before noncardiac surgery (class I, level B)

- Unstable coronary syndromes
- Decompensated heart failure
- Significant arrhythmia
- Severe valvular disease

Adapted from Fleisher LA, Fleischmann KE, Auerbach AD, et al. 2014 ACC/AHA guideline on perioperative cardiovascular evaluation and management of patients undergoing noncardiac surgery: executive summary: a report of the American College of Cardiology/American Heart Association Task Force on practice guidelines. Circulation 2014;130(24):2215–45.

subsequent dementia, and lack of detection worsens outcomes.[25] The Confusion Assessment Method (CAM) is a validated screening tool[26] and has been used in prospective studies to diagnose delirium in patients with hip fracture in the perioperative phase.[27] Please see the article by Inouye SK and colleagues for the Confusion Assessment Method at: https://protect-au.mimecast.com/s/ZXg6BmSwVe6xT1?domain=annals.org. Those patients who do not have delirium diagnosed after assessment with the CAM could undergo further cognitive assessment with tools such as the standardized mini-mental state examination.[28] However, the need for further cognitive assessment may be outweighed by greater clinical priorities. Important others, such as family members, should be offered the opportunity to provide collateral cognitive history on the patient. Tools such as the Informant Questionnaire on Cognitive Decline in the Elderly have been applied in cognitive studies on patients with hip fracture[29] and are a useful supplement to the cognitive collateral history.

Physical examination and pain

The preoperative physical examination involves examination of the affected limb and exploration for signs of other trauma because additional injuries may be masked by delirium and distracting hip pain. The vital signs should be closely monitored and any abnormalities corrected as physiologic abnormalities are associated with intraoperative and postoperative complications (**Table 1**).[30]

The classic presentation of external rotation and shortening and abduction of the affected limb is not evident in all patients and is typically absent in patients with undisplaced fracture.[1] Pain may be elicited with internal or external rotation of the affected limb or with an axial load to the extremity.

The physical examination also includes assessing for signs of dehydration, hypovolemia, and decompensated chronic disease. The skin should be thoroughly examined for pressure or at-risk areas.

Careful attention is given to the pain that the patient is experiencing because inappropriate pain control favors delirium, and those with delirium may receive inadequate analgesia.[20] Early assessment for and administration of opioid analgesia should be undertaken. Nerve blocks of the obturator, lateral cutaneous nerves, and fascia iliaca can be undertaken in the emergency department and may reduce postoperative pain and delirium.[31]

Table 1
Key vital signs and abnormal parameters in hip fracture

	Minor abnormalities[a]	Major abnormalities[b]
Blood pressure in mm Hg	Systolic >180, diastolic >110	Systolic <91
Heart rate and rhythm (beats per minute)	Atrial fibrillation (AF) or supraventricular tachycardia (SVT) 101–120; sinus tachycardia >120, or heart rate (HR) 46–50	AF or SVT >120; ventricular tachycardia; 3rd-degree heart block or HR <46
Temperature (T)	T >38.4 C	T <35°C or T >38.4°C with clinical pneumonia
Oxygenation and carbon dioxide (CO_2)	46 mm Hg < P_{CO_2} <55 mm Hg	Oximetry <90%; P_{O_2} <60 mm Hg; or P_{CO_2} >54 mm Hg

[a] Minor = mildly abnormal but less likely to require correction before surgery.
[b] Major = markedly abnormal and more likely to require correction before surgery.
Adapted from McLaughlin MA, Orosz GM, Magaziner J, et al. Preoperative status and risk of complications in patients with hip fracture. J Gen Int Med 2006;21(3):220; with permission.

Nutrition

Nearly half of older patients with hip fracture are malnourished on hospital presentation.[32] Malnutrition is a contributory factor to hip fracture in older patients[33] and is closely associated with frailty and prefrailty.[34] Postoperatively, adequate nutrition is associated with fewer complications, faster recovery, and reduced hospital stay.[33] Given the requirements for fasting preoperatively, close attention must be paid to nutritional intake, particularly in vulnerable patients with cognitive impairment. The Mini Nutritional Assessment (MNA) is a validated screening tool for older persons and takes less than 10 minutes to complete.[35–37] It may be useful to identify at-risk patients in the preoperative period. The MNA comprises the following 4 parts:

- Anthropometric measurements
- General status
- Dietary information
- Subjective assessment.[36]

Surgical risk

There are many validated surgical risk screening tools,[38–41] but none consider the subtle physiologic characteristics of the older patient.[42] The American Society of Anesthesiology Physical Performance Status (ASA PS) (**Table 2**)[43] is a simple tool used to predict surgical risk and mortality and has been applied in studies on older patients with hip fracture.[44,45] Those with an ASA grade of 3 or 4 are at 44% higher risk of death at 1 year when compared with those of ASA grade 2 or less.[45]

Comorbidities and frailty

More than one-third of the older population with hip fracture have at least one major comorbidity,[46] and the prevalence of comorbidities among patients with hip fracture is increasing.[47] Comorbid profile is a superior predictor of mortality than age in the older population with hip fracture[48] and should be carefully considered in the preoperative assessment. Multiple comorbidity assessment scores have been proposed and applied in clinical research but have not undergone external validation.[20] The Charlson Comorbidity Index (CCI)[49] calculates a survival-based prediction by assigning different weight to a range of comorbidities. The CCI has been applied in outcome studies on older patients with hip fractures, and a meta-analysis revealed that a score of zero conferred a 41% lower risk of death compared with those with a CCI of one or greater.[45]

The coexistence of frailty in older patients with hip fractures should be considered given its high prevalence in the geriatric population[50] and usefulness as a predictor of

Table 2	
American Society of Anesthesiology physical performance status	
Classification	**Definition**
ASA I	A normal healthy patient
ASA II	A patient with mild systemic disease
ASA III	A patient with severe systemic disease
ASA IV	A patient with severe systemic disease that is a constant threat to life
ASA V	A moribund patient who is not expected to survive without the operation
ASA VI	A declared brain-dead patient whose organs are being removed for donor purposes

Adapted from Dripps R. New classification of physical status. Anesthesiology 1963;24:111. Last approved by the ASA House of Delegates on October 15, 2014; is reprinted with permission of the American Society of Anesthesiologists, 1061 American Lane, Schaumburg, Illinois 60173–4973.

surgical outcomes.[51] Many frailty scales are available; however, 2 scales have recently been determined as effective in risk-stratifying preoperative patients and predicting functional outcomes: the National Surgical Quality Improvement Program modified Frailty Index[51,52] and the Reported Edmonton Frail Scale.[53,54]

Medication review

Polypharmacy, defined as the use of more medications than is medically necessary,[55] is present in approximately 50% of older adults.[56] Polypharmacy increases the risk of falls and hip fractures[57–59] and complicates perioperative management of older patients with hip fracture. The preoperative medication assessment should include the following:

- Identification and cessation of any unnecessary or harmful medications
- Identification and rationalization of medications increasing risk of falls
- The recognition of medications required for treating active conditions
- Plan for insulin and diabetes management
- Pain and bowel management plan
- Antithrombotic and anticoagulant management plan

Approximately 62% of older patients with hip fracture are on antithrombotic or anticoagulant treatment at the time of fracture.[60] Structured plans are required for the management of these medications to minimize the risk of bleeding, transfusion, thromboembolic phenomena, and mortality.[61] Although previous use of aspirin is not a contraindication for surgery, the risk associated with clopidogrel remains controversial. However, a recent meta-analysis reported that these patients can be managed by normal protocols with early surgery. The investigators concluded that operating early on patients on clopidogrel is safe and does not appear to confer any clinically significant bleeding risk.[62]

The new oral anticoagulants present a unique challenge in preoperative management because monitoring parameters are not available. For patients on Coumadin, among several algorithms, the one proposed by Wendl-Soeldner and colleagues[62] practically outlines the management of antithrombotic or anticoagulant treatment in the older patient with hip fracture (**Fig. 1**).

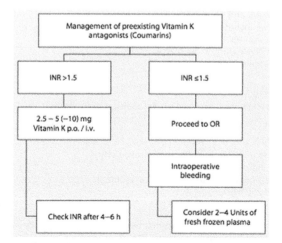

Fig. 1. Management of preexisting vitamin K antagonists (Coumarins). INR, international normalized ratio; i.v., intravenously; OR, operating room; p.o., orally.

Patients undergoing hip fracture surgery should receive thromboembolic prophylaxis at least 12 hours before surgery to reduce the risk of venous thromboembolic phenomena.[63] No difference in bleeding rates was observed between low-molecular-weight heparin or unfractionated heparin.[64] Prophylactic antibiotics, cefazolin 1 g or 2 g, or vancomycin (if beta-lactam allergy), should be administered up to 2 hours before surgery to reduce risk of Staphylococcus aureus infection.[65,66]

Investigations

Preoperative investigations should seek to rapidly confirm the diagnosis of hip fracture, assess the status of comorbidities, increase understanding of the cause of the fall, and expedite postoperative interventions such as osteoporosis treatment. All investigations should be undertaken with the knowledge that a painful or protracted investigatory process may increase distress and the risk of delirium and may cause unnecessary surgical delay. Box 2 outlines the key preoperative investigations in addition to investigations that may contribute to etiological investigation and postoperative management.

An abnormal preoperative electrocardiogram (ECG) is an independent predictor of mortality in patients with hip fracture[45] and should be routinely performed in elevated-risk procedures such as hip fracture surgery.[19] Subsequent cardiac investigations would be dependent on the clinical history, ECG findings, and clinical examination. In the case of significant arrhythmia, cardiac monitoring may be required. Echocardiography is generally not required for decompensated cardiac failure, but may be considered where severe valvular

---

Box 2
Preoperative investigations (excluding hip imaging)

Required for preoperative assessment
  Full blood count (FBC)[a,b]
  Electrolytes[a]
  Blood urea nitrogen[a]
  Calcium, magnesium, and phosphate
  Coagulation profile including international normalized ratio[a]
  Glucose liver function tests including albumin
  Blood group, antibodies, and cross-match
  Chest radiograph/plain radiograph
  ECG

Investigations to consider
  To assist with determining falls cause or metabolic abnormalities
    Vitamin B12
    Red cell folate
    Thyroid function
    Midstream urine microscopy, culture, and sensitivity
    Iron studies (if indicated on FBC)
  To assist with postoperative osteoporosis management
    Vitamin D level 25(OH)D$_3$
    Parathyroid hormone

  [a] Denotes investigations in which abnormalities confer increased odds of cardiopulmonary and postoperative complications in patients with hip fracture.[30]
  [b] Refers to the hemoglobin as a subset of the full blood count.

abnormality is suspected.[20] Practice guidelines on perioperative cardiovascular evaluation are available from the American College of Cardiology/American Heart Association.[19]

Preoperative anemia
The World Health Organization defines anemia as a hemoglobin level of less than 130 g/L in men and less than 120 g/L in women.[67] Preoperative anemia is present in 35% to 53% of older patients with hip fracture.[68] In the general population, preoperative anemia is associated with an increased risk of cardiac events, pneumonia, delirium, mortality, and blood transfusion.[69–71] A randomized controlled trial in high-risk patients with hip fracture found that a liberal (hemoglobin, Hb <10 g/L) transfusion strategy, compared with a restrictive strategy (Hb <8 g/L), did not reduce mortality risk, inability to walk at 60-day follow-up, or in-hospital complications.[72] It is to be noted that this was a study on postoperative anemia, and the precise targets in the preoperative patient remain unclear.

Imaging
Plain film radiography remains the first imaging investigation in patients suspected of hip fracture. Initial radiographs are not confirmatory of hip fracture in 2% to 10% of patients that subsequently have the diagnosis of hip fracture confirmed.[73] Severe osteopenia may mask fracture transparency and sensitivity of plain radiography.[74] Should plain film radiography not identify a hip fracture for a patient in whom significant clinical suspicion exists or where there is concern of possible metastases, osteonecrosis, or Paget disease contributing to the fracture, MRI, computed tomography (CT), and bone scintigraphy are to be considered.[74] MRI is generally considered the reference technique and gold standard.[74,75]

Diagnostic delay of hip fracture can lead to avascular necrosis, nonunion, increased pain and mortality risk, and greater risk of thromboembolic complications.[76,77] The decision on the preferred modality may depend on clinical and operative aims, suspicion for alternative abnormality, timeliness, patient claustrophobia, and resource availability.[78] Access to any modality should not cause a delay in diagnosis and treatment.[78,79] **Fig. 2** outlines an imaging decision tree, and **Table 3** compares the features of different imaging modalities in hip fracture.

Preoperative indicators of mortality and morbidity
The strongest preoperative indicators of postoperative mortality in hip fracture are prefracture mobility, age, abnormal ECG, and cognitive impairment.[45] The summary of a meta-analysis with relative risk of mortality at 12 months following hip fracture is summarized in **Table 4**.

In addition to being a useful predictor of mortality in hip fracture, higher ASA class is strongly associated with postoperative complications and morbidity,[85] although it is not predictive of functional outcome.[86] The MNA in short form is a useful tool in predicting functional outcomes, with malnutrition and risk of malnutrition predictive of institutionalization, and risk of malnutrition predictive of mobility decline at 4 months after fracture.[87] A systematic review of preoperative indicators for postoperative morbidity was not available in the examined literature, and future studies are needed to further establish such indicators.

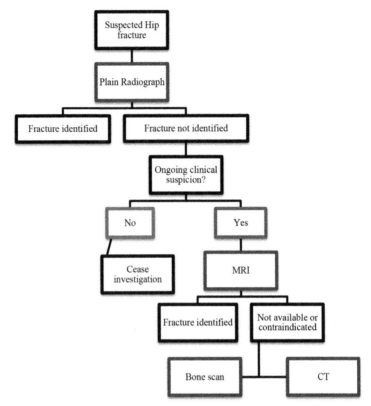

Fig. 2. Decision tree for imaging in suspected hip fracture. (*Adapted from* National Clinical Guideline Center (UK). The Management of Hip Fracture in Adults. London: Royal College of Physicians (UK); 2011. (NICE Clinical Guidelines, No. 124.) 5, Imaging options in occult hip fracture. Available at: http://www.ncbi.nlm.nih.gov/books/NBK83026/ and www.imaging pathways.health.wa.gov.au. Accessed August 28, 2016; with permission; and Government of Western Australia. Diagnostic imaging pathways—hip fracture (suspected). Diagnostic Imaging Pathways. vol. 2016: Government of Western Australia, 2013.)

Table 3				
Comparison of imaging modalities for hip fracture				
Modality				
Feature	**Plain Film**	**CT**	**MRI**	**Bone Scintigraphy**
Cost	Low[79]	Intermediate[79]	High[79]	High[79]
Time	<3 min	<5 min	<10 min	Start >24 h, 4 h for image
Sensitivity	90%–98%[79]	70%–95%[80,81]	100%[82]	75%–98%[83]
Specificity	No evidence	No evidence	100%[82]	100%[83]
Contrast	N/A	Available	Available	Required
Other		3D reconstruction, informs surgical approach. Does not show bone edema	Early detection of oedema in fracture. No radiation Contraindications	Examines whole skeleton
Radiation[84]	++ to +++	+++ to ++++	N/A	+++

Abbreviations: 3D, 3-dimensional; N/A, not applicable.

Table 4
Preoperative characteristics and mortality risk 12 months following hip fracture

Outcome	Relative Risk	P Value
Gender (F:M)	0.68 (0.62, 0.76)	<.0001
Age (< vs ≥85 y)	0.42 (0.20, 0.90)	.0009
CCI (0 vs 1+)	0.59 (0.56, 0.61)	<.0001
Residence (home vs institution)	0.57 (0.43, 0.72)	.01
Fracture type (intracapsular vs extracapsular)	0.77 (0.63, 0.95)	<.0001
ASA grade (1 or 2 vs 3 or 4)	0.44 (0.35, 0.56)	<.0001
Cognitive impairment	1.91 (1.35, 2.70)	.0002
Mobility (independent vs require assistance)	0.13 (0.05, 0.34)	<.0001
Abnormal ECG	2.00 (1.45, 2.76)	<.001

Adapted from Smith T, Pelpola K, Ball M, et al. Pre-operative indicators for mortality following hip fracture surgery: a systematic review and meta-analysis. Age Aging 2014;43(4):464–71; with permission.

SUMMARY

Considering that nearly 50% of patients with hip fracture will develop at least one short-term complication during the postoperative period, prompt identification of the potential complications, it is hoped during the preoperative assessment, is pivotal. Short-term postoperative complications (first 30–90 days) include infection, delirium, venous thromboembolism, pressure ulcers, or cardiovascular events. Most of these events could be predicted by a comprehensive preoperative assessment.

In terms of long-term complications (between 90 days and 1 year after surgery), which include disability, falls, secondary fractures, and mortality, a comprehensive assessment should also be able to predict these complications. For instance, high ASA scale and prior inability to ambulate are stronger predictors of short-term complications and poor outcomes. More than 50% of previously independent patients develop a new requirement for assistance with lower extremity functional tasks or instrumental ADL. To prevent further disability, a complete identification of the baseline functional status is pivotal. Strong predictors of mortality include advanced age, male gender, nursing home residence, poor preoperative walking capacity, poor ADL, higher ASA grading, multiple comorbidities, dementia or cognitive impairment, diabetes, cancer, and cardiac disease. All these predictors could also be identified in the preoperative period. Interestingly, hip fractures have been associated with higher mortality due to cardiovascular events even in patients without previous history of cardiovascular disease. This complication could be prevented by prompt administration of osteoporosis treatment in previously untreated patients.[88]

In conclusion, a comprehensive geriatric assessment, combined with a battery of imaging and blood tests, should be able to identify those patients with hip fracture who are at higher risk of short- and long-term complications. This comprehensive assessment should be followed by the implementation of a comprehensive multidimensional care plan aimed to prevent negative outcomes in the postoperative period (short and long term), thus assuring a safe and prompt functional recovery while also preventing future falls and fractures.

REFERENCES

1. LeBlanc K, Muncie H, LeBlanc L. Hip fracture: diagnosis, treatment, and secondary prevention. Am Fam Physician 2014;89(12):945–51.

2. Auron-Gomez M, Michota F. Medical management of hip fracture. Clin Geriatr Med 2008;24(4):701–19.
3. Campbell M, Fitzpatrick R, Haines A, et al. Framework for design and evaluation of complex interventions to improve health. BMJ 2000;321(7262):694–6.
4. Campbell NC, Murray E, Darbyshire J, et al. Designing and evaluating complex interventions to improve health care. BMJ 2007;334(7591):455–9.
5. Panella M, Marchisio S, Di Stanislao F. Reducing clinical variations with clinical pathways: do pathways work? Int J Qual Health Care 2003;15(6):509–21.
6. Leigheb F, Vanhaecht K, Sermeus W, et al. The effect of care pathways for hip fractures: a systematic review. Calcif Tissue Int 2012;91(1):1–14.
7. Lee DJ, Elfar JC. Timing of hip fracture surgery in the elderly. Geriatr Orthop Surg Rehabil 2014;5(3):138–40.
8. Bottle A, Aylin P. Mortality associated with delay in operation after hip fracture: observational study. BMJ 2006;332(7547):947–51.
9. Uzoigwe CE, Burnand HG, Cheesman CL, et al. Early and ultra-early surgery in hip fracture patients improves survival. Injury 2013;44(6):726–9.
10. Al-Ani AN, Samuelsson B, Tidermark J, et al. Early operation on patients with a hip fracture improved the ability to return to independent living. A prospective study of 850 patients. J Bone Joint Surg Am 2008;90(7):1436–42.
11. Doruk H, Mas MR, Yildiz C, et al. The effect of the timing of hip fracture surgery on the activity of daily living and mortality in elderly. Arch Gerontol Geriatr 2004; 39(2):179–85.
12. Grimes JP, Gregory PM, Noveck H, et al. The effects of time-to-surgery on mortality and morbidity in patients following hip fracture. Am J Med 2002;112(9): 702–9.
13. Majumdar SR, Beaupre LA, Johnston DW, et al. Lack of association between mortality and timing of surgical fixation in elderly patients with hip fracture: results of a retrospective population-based cohort study. Med Care 2006;44(6):552–9.
14. Moran CG, Wenn RT, Sikand M, et al. Early mortality after hip fracture: is delay before surgery important? J Bone Joint Surg Am 2005;87(3):483–9.
15. Hapuarachchi KS, Ahluwalia RS, Bowditch MG. Neck of femur fractures in the over 90s: a select group of patients who require prompt surgical intervention for optimal results. J Orthop Traumatol 2014;15(1):13–9.
16. Shiga T, Wajima Z, Ohe Y. Is operative delay associated with increased mortality of hip fracture patients? Systematic review, meta-analysis, and meta-regression. Can J Anaesth 2008;55(3):146–54.
17. Moja L, Piatti A, Pecoraro V, et al. Timing matters in hip fracture surgery: patients operated within 48 hours have better outcomes. A meta-analysis and meta-regression of over 190,000 patients. PLoS one 2012;7(10):e46175.
18. Simunovic N, Devereaux PJ, Sprague S, et al. Effect of early surgery after hip fracture on mortality and complications: systematic review and meta-analysis. CMAJ 2010;182(15):1609–16.
19. Fleisher LA, Fleischmann KE, Auerbach AD, et al. 2014 ACC/AHA guideline on perioperative cardiovascular evaluation and management of patients undergoing noncardiac surgery: executive summary: a report of the American College of Cardiology/American Heart Association task force on practice guidelines. Circulation 2014;130(24):2215–45.
20. Boddaert J, Raux M, Khiami F, et al. Perioperative management of elderly patients with hip fracture. Anesthesiology 2014;121(6):1336–41.
21. Freter S, Dunbar M, Koller K, et al. Prevalence and characteristics of preoperative delirium in hip fracture patients. Gerontology 2016;62(4):396–400.

22. Ambrose AF, Cruz L, Paul G. Falls and fractures: a systematic approach to screening and prevention. Maturitas 2015;82(1):85–93.
23. Rosell PA, Parker MJ. Functional outcome after hip fracture. A 1-year prospective outcome study of 275 patients. Injury 2003;34(7):529–32.
24. Inouye SK. Predisposing and precipitating factors for delirium in hospitalized older patients. Dement Geriatr Cogn Disord 1999;10(5):393–400.
25. Krogseth M, Wyller TB, Engedal K, et al. Delirium is an important predictor of incident dementia among elderly hip fracture patients. Dement Geriatr Cogn Disord 2011;31(1):63–70.
26. Inouye SK, van Dyck CH, Alessi CA, et al. Clarifying confusion: the confusion assessment method. A new method for detection of delirium. Ann Intern Med 1990;113(12):941–8.
27. Watne LO, Torbergsen AC, Conroy S, et al. The effect of a pre- and postoperative orthogeriatric service on cognitive function in patients with hip fracture: randomized controlled trial (Oslo Orthogeriatric Trial). BMC Med 2014;12:63.
28. Folstein MF, Folstein SE, McHugh PR. "Mini-mental state". A practical method for grading the cognitive state of patients for the clinician. J Psychiatr Res 1975; 12(3):189–98.
29. Jorm AF. A short form of the informant questionnaire on cognitive decline in the elderly (IQCODE): development and cross-validation. Psychol Med 1994;24(1): 145–53.
30. McLaughlin MA, Orosz GM, Magaziner J, et al. Preoperative status and risk of complications in patients with hip fracture. J Gen Intern Med 2006;21(3):219–25.
31. Rashiq S, Vandermeer B, Abou-Setta AM, et al. Efficacy of supplemental peripheral nerve blockade for hip fracture surgery: multiple treatment comparison. Can J anaesthesian 2013;60(3):230–43.
32. Akner G, Cederhol T. Treatment of protein-energy malnutrition in chronic non-malignant disorders. Am J Clin Nutr 2001;74:6–24.
33. Hedström M, Ljungqvist O, Cederholm T. Metabolism and catabolism in hip fracture patients: nutritional and anabolic intervention—a review. Acta Orthop 2006; 77(5):741–7.
34. Bollwein J, Volkert D, Diekmann R, et al. Nutritional status according to the mini nutritional assessment (MNA®) and frailty in community dwelling older persons: a close relationship. J Nutr Health Aging 2013;17(4):351–6.
35. Vellas B, Guigoz Y, Garry PJ, et al. The mini nutritional assessment (MNA) and its use in grading the nutritional state of elderly patients. Nutrition 1999;15(2): 116–22.
36. Guigoz Y, Vellas B, Garry P. Mini nutritional assessment. A practical assessment tool for grading the nutritional status of elderly patients. Facts Res Gerontol 1994; 4(suppl 2):15–59.
37. Guigoz Y. The mini nutritional assessment (MNA) review of the literature–what does it tell us? J Nutr Health Aging 2006;10(6):466–85 [discussion: 485–7].
38. Gupta PK, Franck C, Miller WJ, et al. Development and validation of a bariatric surgery morbidity risk calculator using the prospective, multicenter NSQIP dataset. J Am Coll Surg 2011;212(3):301–9.
39. Lee TH, Marcantonio ER, Mangione CM, et al. Derivation and prospective validation of a simple index for prediction of cardiac risk of major noncardiac surgery. Circulation 1999;100(10):1043–9.
40. Fleisher LA, Beckman JA, Brown KA, et al. ACC/AHA 2007 guidelines on perioperative cardiovascular evaluation and care for noncardiac surgery: executive summary: a report of the American College of Cardiology/American Heart

Association task force on practice guidelines (writing committee to revise the 2002 guidelines on perioperative cardiovascular evaluation for noncardiac surgery) developed in collaboration with the American Society of Echocardiography, American Society of Nuclear Cardiology, Heart Rhythm Society, Society of Cardiovascular Anesthesiologists, Society for Cardiovascular Angiography and Interventions, Society for Vascular Medicine and Biology, and Society for Vascular Surgery. J Am Coll Cardiol 2007;50(17):1707–32.

41. Qaseem T. Risk assessment for and strategies to reduce perioperative pulmonary complications. Ann Intern Med 2006;145(7):553.

42. Kim S, Brooks AK, Groban L. Preoperative assessment of the older surgical patient: honing in on geriatric syndromes. Clin Interv Aging 2015;10:13–27.

43. Dripps R. New classification of physical status. Anesthesiology 1963;24:111.

44. Pereira SR, Puts MT, Portela MC, et al. The impact of prefracture and hip fracture characteristics on mortality in older persons in Brazil. Clin Orthop Relat Res 2010; 468(7):1869–83.

45. Smith T, Pelpola K, Ball M, et al. Pre-operative indicators for mortality following hip fracture surgery: a systematic review and meta-analysis. Age Ageing 2014;43(4): 464–71.

46. Roche JJ, Wenn RT, Sahota O, et al. Effect of comorbidities and postoperative complications on mortality after hip fracture in elderly people: prospective observational cohort study. Br Med J 2005;331(7529):1374.

47. Brauer CA, Coca-Perraillon M, Cutler DM, et al. Incidence and mortality of hip fractures in the United States. JAMA 2009;302(14):1573–9.

48. Graver A, Merwin S, Collins L, et al. Comorbid profile rather than age determines hip fracture mortality in a nonagenarian population. HSS J 2015;11(3):223–35.

49. Charlson ME, Pompei P, Ales KL, et al. A new method of classifying prognostic comorbidity in longitudinal studies: development and validation. J Chronic Dis 1987;40(5):373–83.

50. Handforth C, Clegg A, Young C, et al. The prevalence and outcomes of frailty in older cancer patients: a systematic review. Ann Oncol 2015;26(6):1091–101.

51. Dayama A, Olorunfemi O, Greenbaum S, et al. Impact of frailty on outcomes in geriatric femoral neck fracture management: an analysis of national surgical quality improvement program dataset. Int J Surg 2016;28:185–90.

52. Velanovich V, Antoine H, Swartz A, et al. Accumulating deficits model of frailty and postoperative mortality and morbidity: its application to a national database. J Surg Res 2013;183(1):104–10.

53. Hilmer SN, Perera V, Mitchell S, et al. The assessment of frailty in older people in acute care. Australas J Ageing 2009;28(4):182–8.

54. Kua J, Ramason R, Rajamoney G, et al. Which frailty measure is a good predictor of early post-operative complications in elderly hip fracture patients? Arch Orthop Trauma Surg 2016;136(5):639–47.

55. Tjia J, Velten SJ, Parsons C, et al. Studies to reduce unnecessary medication use in frail older adults: a systematic review. Drugs Aging 2013;30(5):285–307.

56. Maher RL, Hanlon JT, Hajjar ER. Clinical consequences of polypharmacy in elderly. Expert Opin Drug Saf 2014;13(1):57–65.

57. Fletcher PC, Berg K, Dalby DM, et al. Risk factors for falling among community-based seniors. J Patient Saf 2009;5(2):61–6.

58. Garcia O, Jimenez R, Velasco J, et al. Polypharmacy related with increased risk of hip fracture in the older patients. Eur J Hosp Pharm Sci Pract 2012;19(2):107.

59. Damian J, Pastor-Barriuso R, Valderrama-Gama E, et al. Factors associated with falls among older adults living in institutions. BMC Geriatr 2013;13:6.

60. Bucking B, Bliemel C, Waschnick L, et al. Anticoagulation medication for proximal femoral fractures: prospective validation study of new institutional guidelines. Unfallchirurg 2013;116(10):909–15.

61. Wendl-Soeldner MA, Moll CW, Kammerlander C, et al. Algorithm for anticoagulation management in geriatric hip fracture patients–surgeons save blood. Z Gerontol Geriatr 2014;47(2):95–104.

62. Soo CG, Torre PKD, Yolland TJ, et al. Clopidogrel and hip fractures, is it safe? A systematic review and meta-analysis. BMC Musculoskelet Disord 2016;17:136.

63. Holbrook A, Schulman S, Witt DM, et al. Evidence-based management of anticoagulant therapy: antithrombotic therapy and prevention of thrombosis, 9th ed: American College of Chest Physicians evidence-based clinical practice guidelines. Chest 2012;141(2 Suppl):e152S–84S.

64. Handoll HH, Farrar MJ, McBirnie J, et al. Heparin, low molecular weight heparin and physical methods for preventing deep vein thrombosis and pulmonary embolism following surgery for hip fractures. Cochrane Database Syst Rev 2000;(2):CD000305.

65. Bratzler DW, Dellinger EP, Olsen KM, et al. Clinical practice guidelines for antimicrobial prophylaxis in surgery. Surg Infect 2013;14(1):73–156.

66. Gillespie WJ, Walenkamp GH. Antibiotic prophylaxis for surgery for proximal femoral and other closed long bone fractures. Cochrane Database Syst Rev 2010;(3):CD000244.

67. WHO/UNICEF/UNU. Iron deficiency anaemia assessment, prevention, and control: a guide for programme managers. Geneva (Switzerland): World Health Organization; 2001.

68. Spahn DR. Anemia and patient blood management in hip and knee surgery: a systematic review of the literature. Anesthesiology 2010;113(2):482–95.

69. Goodnough LT, Maniatis A, Earnshaw P, et al. Detection, evaluation, and management of preoperative anaemia in the elective orthopaedic surgical patient: NATA guidelines. Br J Anaesth 2011;106(1):13–22.

70. Kumar A. Perioperative management of anemia: limits of blood transfusion and alternatives to it. Cleve Clin J Med 2009;76(Suppl 4):S112–8.

71. Wu WC, Schifftner TL, Henderson WG, et al. Preoperative hematocrit levels and postoperative outcomes in older patients undergoing noncardiac surgery. JAMA 2007;297(22):2481–8.

72. Carson JL, Terrin ML, Noveck H, et al. Liberal or restrictive transfusion in high-risk patients after hip surgery. N Engl J Med 2011;365(26):2453–62.

73. Lubovsky O, Liebergall M, Mattan Y, et al. Early diagnosis of occult hip fractures MRI versus CT scan. Injury 2005;36(6):788–92.

74. Masciocchi C, Conchiglia A, Conti L, et al. Imaging of insufficiency fractures. In: Guglielmi G, Peh W, Guermazi A, editors. Geriatric imaging. Berlin: Springer-Verlag; 2013. p. 83–91.

75. Collin D, Geijer M, Göthlin JH. Computed tomography compared to magnetic resonance imaging in occult or suspect hip fractures. A retrospective study in 44 patients. Eur Radiol 2016;11:1–7.

76. Verbeeten KM, Hermann KL, Hasselqvist M, et al. The advantages of MRI in the detection of occult hip fractures. Eur Radiol 2005;15(1):165–9.

77. Gill SK, Smith J, Fox R, et al. Investigation of occult hip fractures: the use of CT and MRI. ScientificWorldJournal 2013;2013:4.

78. Rehman H, Clement RG, Perks F, et al. Imaging of occult hip fractures: CT or MRI? Injury 2016;47(6):1297–301.

79. National Clinical Guideline Centre (UK). The management of hip fracture in adults [internet]. London: National Clinical Guideline Centre; 2011. p. 7–33. Available at: www.ncgc.ac.uk. Accessed August 28, 2016.

80. Cabarrus MC, Ambekar A, Lu Y, et al. MRI and ct of insufficiency fractures of the pelvis and the proximal femur. AJR Am J Roentgenol 2008;191(4):995–1001.

81. Dunker D, Collin D, Gothlin JH, et al. High clinical utility of computed tomography compared to radiography in elderly patients with occult hip fracture after low-energy trauma. Emerg Radiol 2012;19(2):135–9.

82. Quinn SF, McCarthy JL. Prospective evaluation of patients with suspected hip fracture and indeterminate radiographs: use of t1-weighted MR images. Radiology 1993;187(2):469–71.

83. Evans P, Wilson C, Lyons K. Comparison of MRI with bone scanning for suspected hip fracture in elderly patients. J Bone Joint Surg Br 1994;76-B(1):158–9.

84. Ward RJ, Weissman BN, Kransdorf MJ, et al. ACR appropriateness criteria acute hip pain-suspected fracture. J Am Coll Radiol 2014;11(2):114–20.

85. Donegan DJ, Gay AN, Baldwin K, et al. Use of medical comorbidities to predict complications after hip fracture surgery in the elderly. J Bone Joint Surg Am 2010; 92(4):807–13.

86. Michel JP, Klopfenstein C, Hoffmeyer P, et al. Hip fracture surgery: is the pre-operative American Society of Anesthesiologists (ASA) score a predictor of functional outcome? Aging Clin Exp Res 2002;14(5):389–94.

87. Nuotio M, Tuominen P, Luukkaala T. Association of nutritional status as measured by the mini-nutritional assessment short form with changes in mobility, institutionalization and death after hip fracture. Eur J Clin Nutr 2016;70(3):393–8.

88. Center JR, Bliuc D, Nguyen ND, et al. Osteoporosis medication and reduced mortality risk in elderly women and men. J Clin Endocrinol Metab 2011;96(4): 1006–14.

Rapid Depression Assessment in Geriatric Patients

George T. Grossberg, MD[a,b,c], David Beck, MD[a],
Syed Noman Y. Zaidi, MD[a,*]

KEYWORDS

- Geriatric • Elderly • Depression • Rating scale • Assessing depression
- Patient Health Questionnaire • Geriatric Depression Scale

KEY POINTS

- Depression is common in geriatric patients with multiple comorbid medical illnesses and is often underdiagnosed and undertreated.
- Initial screening for depression can easily be accomplished in the waiting room.
- The clinical interview remains the gold standard for diagnosing geriatric depression, and it should be done with sensitivity to the privacy, but also the need to get information from a reliable informant.
- Illicit substances and medical conditions may significantly contribute.
- Suicide assessment should be done in a step wise manner.

INTRODUCTION

In the 2013 Global Burden of Disease Study, the second leading cause of years lived with disability was major depressive disorder, both worldwide and in the United States.[1] Among the elderly, the prevalence of depression is estimated to be 14% to 42% among residents in US nursing homes and 1.8% among elderly living in private households.[2] This places a significant burden both on patients, their families, and society. After adjusting for age, sex, and extent of chronic disease, the total health care cost for elderly patients with depression was 47% to 51% higher than elderly patients

Disclosures: None.

[a] Department of Psychiatry and Behavioral Neuroscience, Saint Louis University, 1438 South Grand Boulevard, St Louis, MO 63104, USA; [b] Department of Anatomy and Neurobiology, Saint Louis University, 1438 South Grand Boulevard, St Louis, MO 63104, USA; [c] Division of Geriatric Medicine, Department of Internal Medicine, Dementia, Health Aging, Saint Louis University, 1438 South Grand Boulevard, St Louis, MO 63104, USA
* Corresponding author.
E-mail address: Zaidis@slu.edu

Clin Geriatr Med 33 (2017) 383–391
http://dx.doi.org/10.1016/j.cger.2017.03.007

without depression.[3] Possible reasons for increased spending include symptom amplification, increased rates of medication/medical recommendation nonadherence, decreased functional ability, and a direct impact of depression on the course of medical illness.

Factors significantly associated with either depression or depressive symptoms among the elderly include comorbid chronic medical disorders, cognitive impairment, health-related functional impairment, lack of or loss of close social contacts, and a prior history of depression. Increasing age has not consistently been associated with increasing prevalence of depression, and evidence suggests that any age-related effects on depression are more linked to chronic health problems and functional impairment.[4] Chronic diseases such as stroke, loss of hearing, loss of vision, cardiac disease, and chronic lung disease significantly increase the risk of depression in old age.[5]

SCREENING FOR DEPRESSION
Waiting Room

Patients can be provided a GDS-30/GDS-15 (Geriatric Depression scale) or PHQ-2 and then PHQ-9 (Patient Health Questionnaire) while waiting in the waiting area, Patients can be provided a GDS-30/GDS-15 (Geriatric Depression Scale) or PHQ-2 and then PHQ-9 (Patient Health Questionnaire) while waiting in the waiting area.

The GDS-30 is the most evaluated screening tool in the acute inpatient setting, with cut-off values of 10 or 11 appearing to demonstrate the highest sensitivity.[6] Shorter versions of the GDS-30, such as the GDS-15, GDS-4, or GDS-5, have demonstrated conflicting results across studies.[7,8] While the GDS-30 displayed a sensitivity and specificity among inpatients of 84.2% and 79.3%, respectively, the sensitivity of the GDS-15 across 3 inpatient studies was low (32.2%).[9] Scoring on the GDS 30 inferred as 0 to 9 to be normal, 10 to 19 to be mild depression, and 20 to 30 to be severe depression. GDS-15 is inferred as 0 to 4 to be no depression, 5 to 10 suggestive of a mild depression, and 11+ suggestive of severe depression.

The GDS was found to be a valid measure of mild-to-moderate depressive symptoms in Alzheimer patients with mild-to-moderate dementia.[10] However, Alzheimer patients who disavow cognitive deficits also tend to disavow depressive symptoms, and the GDS should be used with caution in such patients, keeping in mind they may not be accurate reporters of their symptoms.

The PHQ-2[11] is a valid screening tool for major depression in older people but should be followed by a more-comprehensive diagnostic process (ie, PHQ-9).[12] PHQ-9 has 9 items, each of which is scored 0 to 3, providing a 0 to 27 severity score. Scores of 5, 10, 15, and 20 are cutoffs for mild, moderate, moderately severe, and severe depression, respectively. Although its specificity differs by age, sex, and ethnic groups, these differences appear to be of little clinical significance.

Clinical Encounter

During a face-to-face clinical encounter, the clinician needs to be observant, as multiple clues for depression can be obtained with focused history taking. Assessment of geriatric depression can be a difficult at times.[13,14] Late-life depression still remains a challenge and is unfortunately and commonly underdiagnosed and inadequately treated.[15] In the United States, older men and older African Americans and Hispanics are at even greater risk of unrecognized/undiagnosed depression. The public health concerns of ineffectively treated depression in late life will increase over time as the population continues to age.

Elderly patients tend to report more physical symptoms rather than classical depressive symptoms. Stigma of a mental health diagnosis still remains high, and patients tend to under-report their symptoms, although some evidence suggests this trend may be changing in recent times. Differentiating symptoms of depression from neuro-vegetative symptoms caused by comorbid medical illness can be difficult. Elderly men tend to present with atypical symptoms of anger and irritability rather than sadness and depression. Apathy is another common presentation for men. Elderly women on the other hand often present with physical complaints of pain, aching, and irritability (**Box 1**).

Several strategies can be utilized to improve the reliability of diagnosis in this population. First and foremost, privacy and confidentiality should be ensured. Elderly patients may be embarrassed by certain depressive symptoms and deny them if family members are present during the interview. Psychological distress should be normalized. Brief educational statements explaining that depression is a biological illness can mitigate their sense of guilt over having depression. Privacy is especially important when asking about the more psychologically based symptoms of depression and suicidality. On the other hand, detailed collateral information should be obtained from a primary caregiver and close family members, if the patient consents. Again, the patient may minimize his or her symptoms or simply not remember them.

Diagnostic and Statistical Manual of Mental Disorders, Fifth Edition (DSM-5) criterion to diagnose major depressive disorder encompasses having 5 or more symptoms including depressed mood, loss of interest, weight or appetite changes, sleep disturbance, poor energy, feeling that life is not worth living anymore, and poor concentration that should be present for at least a 2-week period.[16] Complete and detailed criteria can be found at https://www.psychiatry.org/psychiatrists/practice/dsm.

Suicidality

Suicide is almost twice as common in elderly individuals as in the general population.[17] Rates of suicide in elderly individuals are elevated almost exclusively in Caucasian men. Among those who attempt suicide, elderly people are most likely to complete the attempt successfully.[18] Emphasis should be placed on obtaining detailed suicidal risk assessment in this vulnerable population. The following risk factors for suicidality should be taken in to account seriously during a clinical interview (eg, prior depression history and history of other mental disorders, previous suicide attempt, social

---

Box 1
Challenges in assessing depression in elderly patients

Sex differences:
- Men: anger, apathy, anhedonia, but not sadness
- Women: somatic symptoms, dysphoria

Over expression of somatic complaints

Minimization of psychological problems

Presence of medical comorbidity
- Symptoms: fatigue, anorexia, insomnia, psychomotor retardation, pain
- Cognitive impairment
- Medication adverse effects

Presence of psychiatric comorbidities

Rationalization by patient, family, and/or caregiver

isolation, physical illness, unemployment, family conflict, family history of suicide, impulsivity, psychosis, incarceration, and hopelessness).

Determination of suicide risk must be done confidentially and sensitively. It is best to have family/caregivers out of the room, as the patient may not want to worry or upset family members, that he or she is having suicidal thoughts. Questions should be asked in a step wise manner. The authors suggest assessing suicidality after assessment of other depressive symptoms (**Box 2**).

Depression with Psychotic Symptoms

Psychotic depression is diagnosed in patients with major depression who have hallucinations or delusional thoughts. The common themes of depressive delusions in elderly are guilt, hypochondriasis, nihilism, persecution, and sometimes jealousy and infidelity.

Psychotic symptoms such as auditory or visual hallucinations, looseness of associations and strange delusions are easy to recognize, and patients presenting with these symptoms should be promptly referred for psychiatric treatment. However, many elderly patients present with atypical or subtle symptoms, which may not be discovered without some investigation. Because of limited time available during the initial visit, screening for psychosis should be focused, concentrating on those patients with a relatively high probability of harboring a psychotic thought process or content. Patients at high risk of psychosis include patients with the diagnosis of major depression, substance abuse or dementia and patients who appear guarded, responding to internal stimuli, suspicious or otherwise disorganized or bizarre during the interview.

Screening questions for psychosis can often follow the transitional inquiries referring to other symptoms previously described by the patient. For example, a depressed patient might be asked the questions in **Box 3** (unpublished data, An examination of the factor structure of the SCI-PANSS by Dudek PT, 2005).

Box 2
Questions assessing suicidality

- Assessment of other depressive symptoms

- Hopelessness:
  - Do you see any future for yourself?
  - Can you see anything positive?
  - Do you have any hope?

- Passive death wish:
  - Do you ever feel life is not worth living?
  - Do you ever want to just give up?
  - Do you ever wish you could just go to sleep and not wake up?
  - Do you hope or pray to die?

- Suicidality:
  - Do you ever think about taking your life?
  - Would you play an active role in bringing about your death ?
  - Do you think of hurting yourself?
  - How often?
  - How long do these thoughts stay in your mind?
  - Do you have a plan? If yes then, what is it?
  - Do you think you would follow through on your plan?
  - When did you first have these thoughts?
  - Have you ever done anything like that before?

Box 3
Questions assessing psychosis

- Hallucinations:
  - Do you have any strange or unusual experiences?
  - Sometimes people tell me that they can hear noises or voices that others can't hear. What about you?
  - If hearing voices:
    - Can you recognize whose voices these are?
    - What do the voices say?
    - Are the voices good or bad?
    - Pleasant or unpleasant?
    - Do the voices interrupt your thinking or your activities?
    - Do they sometimes give you orders or instructions?
  - Do ordinary things sometimes look strange and distorted to you?
  - Do you sometimes have "visions" or see things others can't see?
  - If yes: for example?
    - Do these visions seem very real or lifelike?
    - How often do you have these experiences?

- Delusions:
  - Do you ever feel like someone is after you to hurt you?
  - Do you ever feel like someone is stealing from you?
  - Do you ever feel like someone is trying put thoughts in your mind or trying to control your mind?
  - Do you feel as if you are a bad person or have done something bad in the past?
  - Is there anything really bad going on with your physical body right now?
  - Is your spouse or family doing things you do not approve of or are very upsetting to you?

For a substance-abusing patient, the approach might be to ask "Have drugs ever caused your mind to play tricks on you, like seeing things or having paranoid ideas?" Among substance abusers, psychotic ideation may result from acute intoxication (eg, amphetamine or cocaine abuse), chronic use (eg, alcoholic hallucinosis) or withdrawal (eg, delirium tremens).

One of the better approaches for ascertaining delusional ideation in a patient suspected of active paranoia is to assume the patient's perspective: "Have people been harassing you or trying to harm you?" This communicates sympathy for the patient's perceptions and tends to resolve a guarded attitude.

Medication-Induced Depression

Careful review of scheduled and over-the-counter medications, including supplements and herbal preparations, should be performed at each clinical visit. Substance abuse, intoxication or withdrawal can be a reason for patients to develop sad mood or diminished interest or pleasure in all or almost all activities. Following is a partial list of commonly used medications that may mimic clinical depression.

- Narcotic analgesics/opioids
- Benzodiazepines
- Interferon-alpha
- Steroids
- Anti-Parkinsonian drugs
- β blockers
- Cimetidine
- Clonidine

- Hydralazine
- Estrogens
- Progesterone
- Tamoxifen
- Vinblastine
- Vincristine

Medical Comorbidities

Depression in the elderly can be a result of multiple medical and neurologic disorders. Diagnosis of depression due to a general medical condition can be considered if the patient is exhibiting symptoms of depression or loss of interest in the presence of underlying illness associated with depression.

Cardiac Comorbidities

About 1 of every 4 of individuals who have suffered a myocardial infarction or who are undergoing cardiac catheterization have major depression, and another 25% have minor depression.[19] Approximately half of patients with heart disease and major depression will have had at least 1 previous episode of major depression, and half of those with major depression at the time of cardiac catheterization remain depressed a year after the procedure.

Endocrine Disorders

Several hormonal dysfunctions can mimic, mask, or worsen underlying depression. Careful review and comprehensive laboratory evaluations should be performed to rule out underlying hypothyroidism, hyperthyroidism, hypoparathyroidism, hyperparathyroidism, hypoadrenocorticism, hyperadrenocorticism, or Cushing disease. Clinically, thyroid should always be assessed. Adrenal function is usually determined in a detailed fashion only if there are indications of disease from physical examination, vital signs, or other laboratory findings.

Neurologic or Psychiatric Comorbidities

Indications of depression are often present in individuals with major or mild neurocognitive impairments. The point prevalence of major depression is about 17% in patients with Alzheimer disease.[20] As per newer studies, approximately half of the patients with late-onset depression have generalized cognitive impairment.[21] Symptoms of depression are often precursors of cognitive decline[22] and dementia[23] with senior individuals who have major depression and neurocognitive impairment likely to develop major neurocognitive impairments within a few years of onset of depression.[24,25] Symptoms of depression in early years are also a potential risk factor for disorders of dementia. Major depressive disorders with onset more than 10 years before the diagnosis of dementia[26] and lifetime history of depression[27] are linked with increased risk for Alzheimer disease.

In all elderly patients, cognitive screening should be performed. The Saint Louis University Mental Status examination (SLUMS) can be used as a screening tool for cognitive impairment. The SLUMS is a 30-point screening questionnaire that tests for orientation, memory, attention, and executive functions. Although the SLUMS and MMSE (Mini Mental Status Examination) have comparable sensitivities, the SLUMS is possibly better at detecting mild neurocognitive disorder, which the MMSE failed to detect, but this needs to be further investigated.[28] Unlike the MMSE, the SLUMS is also not copyright protected. More recently, a short SLUMS called rapid cognitive screen assessment tool (10 points) has been validated and published.[29]

Box 4
Medical comorbidities associated with depression

Drugs and toxins: benzodiazepines, opiates, reserpine, alpha-methyldopa, propranolol, cimetidine, and steroids

Illicit substances: cocaine, heroin, primary care physician

Neoplasms: pancreatic, bronchogenic carcinoma, brain tumor, lymphomas

Neurologic disease: stroke, Parkinson disease, Huntington disease, chronic subdural hematoma, temporal lobe epilepsy, multiple sclerosis

Heart diseases: coronary artery disease, myocardial infarction, congestive heart failure, mitral valve prolapse, hypoxia

Metabolic: uremia, hyponatremia, hypokalemia

Vitamin deficiency: pellagra, B12/folate deficiency, vitamin D deficiency, thiamine deficiency

Endocrine: hypo/hyperthyroidism, hyper/hypoparathyroidism, hyper/hypo adrenocortical function, hypogonadism

Miscellaneous: Wilson disease, psoriasis, amyloidosis

Parkinson patients deserve special mention at this point. Suicide risk in Parkinson disease patients is approximately 2 times higher than that in the general population.[30] Case control analysis revealed that male gender, initial severity of motor symptom onset, history of depressive disorder, delusions, any psychiatric disorder, and higher L-dopa dosage were significantly associated with suicide among Parkinson disease patients.

It appears that the link between attention deficit hyperactivity disorder (ADHD) and anxiety/depression remains in place with aging. This suggests that, in clinical practice, directing attention to both in concert may be fruitful. Both ADHD diagnosis and more ADHD symptoms in elderly patients are associated with more anxiety and depressive symptoms cross-sectionally as well as longitudinally. The longitudinal analyses showed that respondents with higher scores of ADHD symptoms reported an increase of depressive symptoms over 6 years, whereas respondents with fewer ADHD symptoms remained stable.[31]

Box 4 provides a summary of substance and medical comorbidities associated with depression.

Once the clinician has taken into consideration all the previously mentioned variables and if the suspicion for depression still remains high, then the St Louis University AM SAD[32] (appetite, mood, sleep, activity, and thoughts of death) questionnaire can be utilized. Frequency of occurrence of each symptom over the prior 2 weeks is quantified as: 0 = never, 1 = 1 day only, and 2 = 2 or more days. The maximum total score is 10. Results show that the cutoff score for mild depression was at 3 to 4, and the cutoff for moderate depression was 6.

REFERENCES

1. Global burden of disease. 2013. Available at: http://www.thelancet.com/pdfs/journals/lancet/PIIS0140-6736(15)60692-4.

2. Djernes JK. Prevalence and predictors of depression in populations of elderly: a review. Acta Psychiatr Scand 2006;113:372–87.

3. Katon WJ, Lin E, Russo J, et al. Increased medical costs of a population-based sample of depressed elderly patients. Arch Gen Psychiatry 2003;60(9):897–903.

4. Roberts RE, Kaplan GA, Shema SJ, et al. Does growing old increase the risk for depression? Am J Psychiatry 1997;154(10):1384–90.

5. Huang CQ, Dong BR, Lu ZC, et al. Chronic diseases and risk for depression in old age: a meta-analysis of published literature. Ageing Res Rev 2010;9(2):131–41.

6. Dennis M, Kadri A, Coffey J. Depression in older people in the general hospital: a systematic review of screening instruments. Age Ageing 2012;41(2):148–54.

7. Rinaldi P, Mecocci P, Benedetti C, et al. Validation of the five-item geriatric depression scale in elderly subjects in three different settings. J Am Geriatr Soc 2003;51(5):694–8.

8. Amadori K, Herrmann E, Püllen RK. Comparison of the 15-item geriatric depression scale (GDS-15) and the GDS-4 during screening for depression in an in-patient geriatric patient group. J Am Geriatr Soc 2011;59(1):171–2.

9. Mitchell AJ, Bird V, Rizzo M, et al. Which version of the geriatric depression scale is most useful in medical settings and nursing homes? Diagnostic validity meta-analysis. Am J Geriatr Psychiatry 2010;18(12):1066–77.

10. Feher EP, Larrabee GJ, Crook TH. Factors attenuating the validity of the geriatric depression scale in a dementia population. J Am Geriatr Soc 1992;40(9):906–9.

11. Li C, Friedman B, Conwell Y, et al. Validity of the patient health questionnaire 2 (PHQ-2) in identifying major depression in older people. J Am Geriatr Soc 2007;55(4):596–602.

12. Löwe B, Unützer J, Callahan CM, et al. Monitoring depression treatment outcomes with the patient health questionnaire-9. Med Care 2004;42(12):1194–201.

13. Espinoza R, Unützer J. Diagnosis and management of late-life depression. In: Roy-Byrne P, Schmader KE, editors. UpToDate. Available at: http://www.uptodate.com/contents/diagnosis-and-management-of-late-life-depression.

14. Almeida OP, Alfonso H, Pirkis J, et al. A practical approach to assess depression risk and to guide risk reduction strategies in later life. Int Psychogeriatr 2011;23(2):280–91.

15. Minino AM, Arias E, Kochanek KD, et al. Final data for 2000. Natl Vital Stat Rep 2002;50:1–119.

16. American Psychiatric Association. Diagnostic and statistical manual of mental disorders. 5th edition. Washington, DC: Author; 2013.

17. Conwell Y, Duberstein PR, Caine ED. Risk factors for suicide in later life. Biol Psychiatry 2002;52:193–204.

18. Van Orden KA, Witte TK, Cukrowicz KC, et al. The interpersonal theory of suicide. Psychol Rev 2010;117(2):575–600.

19. Carney RM, Freedland KE. Depression, mortality, and medical morbidity in patients with coronary heart disease. Biol Psychiatry 2003;54:241–7.

20. Wragg RE, Jeste DV. Overview of depression and psychosis in Alzheimer's disease. Am J Psychiatry 1989;146:577–89.

21. Köhler S, Thomas AJ, Barnett NA, et al. The pattern and course of cognitive impairment in late-life depression. Psychol Med 2010;40:591–602.

22. Yaffe K, Blackwell T, Gore R, et al. Depressive symptoms and cognitive decline in non-demented elderly: a prospective study. Arch Gen Psychiatry 1999;56:425–30.

23. Devanand DP, Sano M, Tang MX, et al. Depressed mood and the incidence of Alzheimer's disease in the elderly living in the community. Arch Gen Psychiatry 1996;53:175–82.

24. Alexopoulos GS, Meyers BS, Young RC, et al. The course of geriatric depression with "reversible dementia": a controlled study. Am J Psychiatry 1993;150:1693–9.

25. Kral VA, Emery OB. Long-term follow-up of depressive pseudodementia of the aged. Can J Psychiatry 1989;34:445–6.
26. Jorm AF. History of depression as a risk factor for dementia: an updated review. Aust N Z J Psychiatry 2001;35:776–81.
27. van Duijn CM, Clayton DG, Chandra V, et al. Interaction between genetic and environmental risk factors for Alzheimer's disease: a reanalysis of case-control studies. Genet Epidemiol 1994;11:539–51.
28. Tariq SH, Tumosa N, Chibnall JT, et al. The Saint Louis University Mental Status (SLUMS) Examination for detecting mild cognitive impairment and dementia is more sensitive than the MiniMentalStatus Examination (MMSE)—a pilot study. Am J Geriatr Psych 2006;14:900–10.
29. Malmstrom TK, Voss VB, Cruz-oliver DM, et al. The rapid cognitive screen (RCS): a point-of-care screening for dementia and mild cognitive impairment. J Nutr Health Aging 2015;19(7):741–4.
30. Lee T, Lee HB, Ahn MH, et al. Increased suicide risk and clinical correlates of suicide among patients with Parkinson's disease. Parkinsonism Relat Disord 2016; 32:102–7.
31. Michielsen M, Comijs HC, Semeijn EJ, et al. The comorbidity of anxiety and depressive symptoms in older adults with attention-deficit/hyperactivity disorder: a longitudinal study. J Affect Disord 2013;148(2–3):220–7.
32. Chakkamparambil B, Chibnall JT, Graypel EA, et al. Development of a brief validated geriatric depression screening tool: the SLU "AM SAD". Am J Geriatr Psychiatry 2015;23(8):780–3.

Dissecting Delirium

Phenotypes, Consequences, Screening, Diagnosis, Prevention, Treatment, and Program Implementation

Joseph H. Flaherty, MD[a],*, Jirong Yue, MD[b],
James L. Rudolph, MD, SM[c,d]

KEYWORDS

- Delirium • Aged • Hospital • Cognitive impairment • Antipsychotics
- Quality improvement • Implementation • Attention

KEY POINTS

- Delirium is characterized by an acute change in attention and awareness that affects all cognitive processing. Rapid screening tools and diagnostic criteria are both important.
- Patients with delirium may present differently and different phenotypes are being recognized as the field evolves.
- Despite the seriousness of the consequences of delirium and the availability of screening tools, it is often ignored by the health care system.
- Even the best studies of antipsychotics for delirium have limitations: most focus on perioperative and intensive care unit populations, and results are mixed.
- Strategies for the implementation of delirium prevention and management programs are as important as the models themselves.

Disclosure Statement: Dr J.L. Rudolph is supported by the VA Health Services Research and Development Center of Innovation in Long Term Services and Supports (CIN 13-419) and the VA QUERI-Geriatrics and Extended Care Partnered Evaluation Center for Community Nursing Homes (PEC 15-465). The views and opinions expressed are those of the author and do not reflect the position or policy of the United States Government or the Department of Veterans Affairs.
[a] Division of Geriatrics, Department of Internal Medicine, Saint Louis University, 1402 South Grand Boulevard, Room M238, St Louis, MO 63104, USA; [b] Department of Geriatrics, West China Hospital, Sichuan University, No. 37, Guo Xue Xiang, Chengdu, Sichuan, China; [c] Center of Innovation in Long Term Services and Support, Providence VAMC, 830 Chalkstone Avenue, Building 32, Providence, RI 02908, USA; [d] School of Public Health, Brown School of Medicine, 1215 S Main Street, Providence, RI 02903, USA
* Corresponding author.
E-mail address: flaherty@slu.edu

INTRODUCTION

The subject of delirium is generally looked upon by the practical physician as one of the most obscure in the chain of morbid phenomena.
— *M.B. Gallway, London Medical Gazette, 1838*

Until recently, clinicians feared delirium or considered it a nuisance. However, delirium is receiving due attention. The field continues to grow well beyond internal medicine and surgery to include pediatrics, emergency medicine, palliative care, and post–acute care. This review is intended for clinicians who care for older patients on medical or surgical hospital wards.

DEFINITION AND PHENOTYPES OF DELIRIUM

The criteria for diagnosis of delirium have recently changed, with some ensuing controversy.[1,2] However, for clinicians, understanding the broader concept of delirium will enhance clinical care, regardless of diagnostic criteria.

The poignant description of delirium as "acute brain failure"[3] stands as one of the more valuable to clinicians. As an illness with underlying causes, delirium may be considered an insult to the brain with failure of basic neurophysiologic mechanisms resulting in a change in mental status. The insult is a stressor to the brain function, which keeps the differential diagnosis and clinical treatment of causes rather broad.

As a syndrome, delirium has many cognitive and behavioral characteristics. Thus, the clinician should recognize that the symptoms of delirium may overlap with other diseases or syndromes that affect the brain, particularly dementia with behavioral and psychological symptoms of dementia (BPSD) or Lewy body dementia.

The phenotype or expression of delirium has historically been categorized as hypoactive, hyperactive, or mixed. As the field of delirium expands, phenotypes are also expanding (**Table 1**). The following are reasons for considering different phenotypic categorical models of delirium:

- Differences in outcomes and different outcomes of importance
- Differences in underlying causes and contributing factors
- Differences in prevention and management strategies and interventions
- Neuropathogenesis might be different

For a clinician in a health care system with an increasing focus on standardization, the temptation is to standardize delirium diagnosis, management, and treatment. This simplistic approach to delirium is challenged in a heterogeneous population with multiple predispositions, insults, and phenotypes.

PREVALENCE AND INCIDENCE

Delirium is common in elderly patients. Prevalence and incidence of delirium vary depending on characteristics of patients, evaluation method, and setting of care (**Table 2**).

CONSEQUENCES

Delirium is associated with short-, intermediate-, and long-term negative health outcomes (**Box 1**). Although historically thought to be reversible, recent outcomes studies suggest that delirium can cause lasting brain injury, such as a decline in cognition, at 3 and 12 months after hospitalization.[4] Duration of delirium was associated with more impairment.[4] Severity of delirium may also be associated with an increased risk of death or nursing home admission.[5]

Table 1
Proposed phenotypic categorical models of delirium

Phenotypic Categorical Model	Explanation
Hypoactive/hyperactive/mixed	Traditional concept describing outward appearance of the patient
Sedative/septic/ hypoxic/metabolic/other	Based mainly on ICU patients; describes underlying (or primary) insult or probable cause of the delirium
Intrinsic/extrinsic	Based on whether cause of delirium is direct insult to the brain or is due to external cause
Postoperative delirium (POD) Postoperative cognitive dysfunction (POCD)	Some confusion/overlap in the literature; sometimes used to mean the same thing (any cognitive impairment after surgery) or distinct (POD = change in the acute period; POCD = change that does not clear over longer period of time)
Emergence delirium (from anesthesia)	Distinct from POD and POCD; occurs after awakening from anesthesia; common in children as well
ICU delirium	Definition depends on location of ICU but caution as some postoperative studies put in this category
Delirium at end of life Terminal restlessness	Delirium at end of life has mostly replaced terminal restlessness in literature; emerging studies
Pediatric delirium	Emerging studies
Subsyndromal delirium	An acute change in cognition that does not meet full criteria for delirium
Persistent delirium or chronic delirium	Controversial area that needs more study
Delirium superimposed on dementia	Delirium in patients with underlying dementia; slower recovery times

Table 2
Rates of delirium based on clinical setting or patient population

Setting/Population	Occurrence[a]	
	Prevalence	Incidence
General medical[73]	18%–35%	11%–14%
Oncology ward[74]	—	18%
Hospice settings[75]	26%–44%	Up to 83%
End of life[76,77]	Up to 85%	
Emergency department[78]	7%–20%	
General surgery[9]	9%–24%	
Neurosurgery[9]	14.9%	
Hepatobiliary surgery[9]	17%	
Acute hip surgery[9]	12.5%–48.1%	
Cardiac surgery[9]	13.5%–50%	
Vascular surgery[9]	29.1%–33%	
ICUs[73]	7%–50%	19%–82%
Nursing home or post–acute care[79]	15.9%	

[a] Occurrence indicated when there is ambiguity or overlap between the measurement of prevalence and incidence.

Box 1
Consequences of delirium

Hospital complications (difficulty cooperating with care, falls, pulling IVs)

Loss of function

Increased institutional care after hospitalization (both skilled nursing facility [SNF] and long term care [LTC])

Poorer outcomes at SNF

Increased hospital stay

Increased mortality

Long-term cognitive impairment (persistent, often subtle, cognitive deficits after delirium)

Posttraumatic stress disorder

Increased mortality

Increased costs

Depression

DESPITE THE MORBIDITY AND MORTALITY, DELIRIUM IS IGNORED BY HEALTH CARE

There is strong evidence that delirium is ignored by the health care system, including health care professionals, health care systems, insurance companies, and research funders:

- Delirium occurs in approximately 25% of older hospitalized patients; health care professionals do not identify delirium in up to 75% of cases,[6,7] and delirium is only coded in 0.2%.[8]
- For 20 years, there has been randomized controlled trial (RCT) evidence that delirium is preventable, yet few systems have implemented systematic delirium prevention.[9]
- Delirium is associated with negative consequences, many of which cost health care systems money.[9] As a result, health systems have a financial incentive to implement delirium screening and prevention.
- Given the impact on nearly 4 million hospitalized older patients annually, the 2016 National Institutes of Health funding of $22 million for delirium is lower than $991 million for dementia and $47 million for incontinence.[10]

DIAGNOSIS AND SCREENING: KEY COGNITIVE PROCESSES FOR DELIRIUM

Astute clinicians need to have a deep understanding of the key cognitive processes of delirium because someone in the care process has to lead others in this area in order to avoid underdiagnosis (and missing an underlying serious illness), overdiagnosis (resulting in a hospitalization or pursuing a workup that may cause more harm than good), and misdiagnosis (eg, mistaking BPSD for delirium). Understanding the cognitive processes can also help clinicians develop the skill of knowing when delirium is improving (stay the course) or not (further workup).

Consciousness

As brain science has developed, there is an improved understanding of the hierarchy of cognitive functions. Cognitive functioning requires consciousness. Consciousness has been defined as the ability to arouse (awaken) and demonstrate awareness (verbally respond to cues). If a person lacks consciousness, such as in a coma, it is not possible to further assess cognitive functions. However, consciousness and its components of arousal and awareness occur on a spectrum and can fluctuate.[2]

Attention

Once a patient is awake and able to receive stimuli, the attentional network consists of 4 key processes that allow the patient to survive in their environment, which are described in **Box 2**. Attention is a complex, but rudimentary function[11] that can be illustrated with a survival example. For example, a person walking in the woods hears a noise (alerting); the visual and auditory sensory functions hone in on the location of the noise (orienting); a large bear is seen in the area of the noise (executive), but it is not threatening and the course of action is to stop and observe (self-regulation).[12] The attentional system is critical to the assessment of all other cognitive functions, and impairment in attention will limit the performance within other cognitive domains. **Box 2** describes the domains of consciousness and attention, with respective actions, and examples of these actions.[13,14]

Delirium Diagnosis

The core cognitive deficit in delirium is an acute disturbance in attention as defined by the Diagnostic and Statistical Manual of Mental Disorders, 5th edition (DSM-5). Attention is a broad cognitive construct including the ability to direct, focus, sustain, and shift cognitive ability.[15] Importantly, the DSM-5 recognizes that patients who are acutely unable to attend due to deficiencies in arousal should be considered as having delirium, because arousal is required for assessment of any cognitive domain.[1] **Box 3** describes the criteria for diagnosis of delirium.

"Rapid" Delirium Screening

Although some experts recommend routine screening for delirium using systematic application of *diagnostic* tools,[16] some are too complex or time consuming for routine application. For example, the high sensitivity and specificity of the confusion assessment method come after standardized cognitive screening,[17] (ie, performing a validated mental status examination that may take10–15 minutes). Health care professionals have limited ability to perform this assessment 3 times daily on a busy clinical ward. When the algorithms are used without cognitive screening, the sensitivity and specificity decline.[18]

For *implementation* of systematic delirium screening, several instruments offer improved clinical applicability and preserve the identification of delirium. The Nursing Delirium Screening Checklist is a rapid delirium nursing screening instrument.[19] The Delirium Observation and Screening Scale is a nursing checklist that is completed

Box 2		
Domains of consciousness and attention, with respective actions, and examples of these actions		
Domain	**Action**	**Example of Action**
Consciousness	Arousal	Awaken
	Awareness	Verbally respond to cues
Attention	Alerting process	Is the information important?
	Orienting	Collect additional information
	Executive function	Recruit additional cognitive domains
	Self-regulation	Make decisions on the information

Box 3
Criteria for diagnosis of delirium based on the Diagnostic and Statistical Manual of Mental Disorders, 5th edition

Inattention	Reduced ability to:
	Direct
	Focus
	Shift
	Sustain
	Inability to engage with interview or cognitive assessment
Reduced awareness	Unable to orient to the environment
	Not coma
Acute onset	Change from baseline
	Fluctuates over course of day
Disturbance in cognition	Memory impairment
	Disorientation
	Language deficit
	Decreased visuospatial abilities
	Perception deficit
Not related to a preexisting neurocognitive deficit	Dementia, especially BPSD
	Lewy body dementia
	Parkinson disease
	Frontotemporal dementia
	Vascular dementia

---

over 3 nursing shifts that captures fluctuation and is easy to incorporate into a medical record.[20] The Recognizing Acute Delirium As Routine consists of 3 observational questions that takes approximately 7 seconds.[21] The 4-Attention Test is an operationalized delirium screening assessment that is being implemented in health care systems across Scotland.[22]

As important as the screening tool is a comprehensive, stepwise implementation strategy (**Box 4**). A critical recognition in implementation is that the local environment has to be evaluated and managed by champions.[23] These champions will serve as the face and voice of the implementation, and choice of these champions is critical. Another important strategy is to have staff interventions for first steps if a patient screens positive for delirium. In this way, staff is invested in the screening program because they can actively contribute.

Screening for Delirium with Arousal: Area of Controversy

The ability to arouse is a basic cognitive process that has a neuroanatomical foundation in the reticular activating system of the brainstem[24] and is a fundamental component of consciousness.[25] Although the DSM-5 delirium criteria have deemphasized arousal, the guidance acknowledges that those patients who are unable to arouse should be judged as having "severe inattention."[15] Effectively, arousal is required for assessment of attention.[12] Therefore, if a patient acutely is unable to arouse sufficiently to complete attention assessment, then he or she has delirium.[1] Recent studies have highlighted the importance of arousal in the diagnosis of delirium[26,27] and the adverse consequences of impaired arousal.[28,29]

CAUSES

Traditionally, clinicians have approached the causes of delirium like other syndromes in medicine, using a differential diagnosis and pursuing laboratory or radiologic tests

---

Box 4
Delirium program implementation checklist

1. Take the pulse of the organization
   Who is interested in delirium?
   Any recent stories of delirium impacting other processes?
   Is there leadership support?

2. Identify alliances
   Falls prevention
   Patient safety
   Risk management
   Accountable care organizations
   Other services (surgery, medicine, anesthesia, intensive care)

3. Identify champions
   Leaders among clinical teams
   Open to new methods

4. Identify the process steps
   Identify what steps are currently being completed
   Which team members are completing the steps?
   How is information communicated?
   Are there gaps in the process?

5. Plan-do-study-act
   Identify target steps for intervention
   Keep narrow focus on actionable steps
   Try a new strategy within the narrow focus
   Evaluate if the new strategy worked
   Why did it work (fail)?
   What needs to change?
   Repeat step 5 with other focused steps

6. Expand beyond initial area
   Begin at step 1

---

based on the patient's complaints or physical examination signs. This approach is limited because often delirious patients cannot give a full history or may not cooperate with the examination, leading to overtesting. Although it is still important to have a quick knowledge of all potential causes or contributors (**Table 3**), and that the causes of delirium are commonly multifactorial, a consideration of phenotype might help the clinician narrow the differential (see **Table 1**).

NEUROPATHOPHYSIOLOGY

Before reviewing pharmacologic prevention and treatment of delirium, it is important to recognize that delirium lacks a single common final pathway that can be "treated" or modified with medication. There are at least 7 proposed neuropathophysiology (NPP) hypotheses that try to explain the "complex behavioral and cognitive changes observed in delirium," including[30]

- Neuroinflammatory hypothesis
- Neuronal aging hypothesis
- Oxidative stress hypothesis
- Neurotransmitter deficiency hypothesis
- Neuroendocrine hypothesis
- Diurnal dysregulation hypothesis
- Network disconnectivity hypotheses

Table 3
Potential causes or contributors to delirium: DELIRIUM IS PAINFUL mnemonic

Cause or Contributor	Comments
D Drugs	Almost any drug can affect mental status in broadest terms, especially in vulnerable brain; maintain high index of suspicion
E Eyes, ears	Impaired vision and hearing are more contributors than causes
L Low 02 insults	Hypoxic insults such as myocardial infarction, pulmonary embolus, stroke
I Infection	Severity of infection is important but even mild infection may cause delirium in vulnerable patient; caution not to "overtreat"
R Retention of urine	Coined "cystocerebral syndrome" in the literature, usually causes sudden delirium, muteness, and restlessness
I Ictal, postictal seizures	Not in initial differential diagnosis unless history suggestive, but absence or partial seizures often missed as cause of delirium
U Underhydration	Dehydration and even underhydration can contribute to delirium
M Metabolic	Electrolyte abnormalities (causes and potential contributors)
I Inactivity	Based on studies that early mobilization can decrease delirium
S Sleep deprivation	Also sleep-wake cycle abnormalities important
P Pain	Delirious patients can be assessed for pain
A Attachments (intravenous lines [IVs], telemetry)	Contributors
I Impaction	Severe constipation
N Neurologic injury	(Subdural hematoma, even trauma to brain without subdural)
F Foley	Not just because of risk of infection but considered a "one-point" restraint and impairs mobility
U Undernutrition	Contributor and potentially related to drug side effects (protein-binding)
L Lights, loud noises	Environmental contributors; patients with delirium can misperceive sensory input

The complexity of delirium does not lie in the 7 NPPs alone; these pathways may coexist and overlap. For the clinician, realizing that none of these mechanisms individually fully explain the symptoms observed in delirium has implications for treatment. Treatment of any NPP pathway with medication, without consideration of other pathways, is likely to be ineffective. Furthermore, even treating one NPP is complex, for example, trying to treat the "neurotransmitter deficiency" with antipsychotics. These medications affect multiple receptor targets at one time (dopamine, muscarinic, histaminic, adrenergic), and thus their effect is unpredictable in delirium.

PHARMACOLOGIC PREVENTION AND TREATMENT OF DELIRIUM

Reviews, textbook chapters, and systematic reviews often come to the conclusion that the evidence for using medications to prevent or treat delirium is too low or insufficient enough to recommend their routine use. However, these same reviews and chapters recommend that medications can or should be reserved for management of symptoms of delirium if the symptoms are bothersome to the patient or put the patient or others at risk for harm. Most also conclude that antipsychotics should be considered first line.[9,16,31,32]

Rather than perpetuate this concept by trying to fit the results of less than optimal studies into what currently is being practiced, this section takes a different approach to the available published studies and answers 3 questions by focusing on the highest-quality studies, namely, double-blind, randomized placebo controlled trials (DB-RPCTs), to help clinicians better understand just where the research is related to pharmacology of delirium and how the research does or does not apply to their patients:

1. What clinical settings have been used for DB-RPCTs, and do these studies include the type of patients I will treat?

   As seen in **Table 4**,[31–33] there is a lack of DB-RPCTS for older medical patients outside the intensive care unit (ICU) and perioperative patient populations. The only DB-RPCT of non-ICU medical inpatients was a treatment study comparing quetiapine with placebo (n = 42). It had rigorous methods. It was well blinded and randomized. However, there were no differences in the groups in resolution of delirium at several time points. Although this study, published in 2010, showed that it is feasible to do a DB-RPCT in this population, studies like this one have not been replicated. Although there are numerous single-drug studies and studies comparing different antipsychotics among medical inpatients, with or without psychiatric consultations, and many studies among palliative care patients, because the natural history of delirium is that it usually improves over time with good care, these studies cannot support the conclusions that they are effective unless there is a true placebo group.

2. If meta-analyses are to be used, are there limitations that are not being identified in the usual methods of a review that clinicians who care for older patients need to be aware of?

   Although meta-analyses have significantly moved the field of evidence-based medicine forward and can save busy clinicians time, there are potential limitations of some of the included studies that geriatric clinicians need to be aware of. Furthermore, it may help clinicians to be aware of these studies because they are used in meta-analyses that appear in geriatric journals.[31] **Table 5** uses 3 frequently cited DB-RPCTs of antipsychotics on prevention[34] and treatment[35,36] of delirium to demonstrate these points.

3. For placebo controlled trials, beyond the usual demographics and basic characteristics, were there differences among patients in the placebo group that could have biased the results of the study?

   Placebo controlled trials are one of the most important types of studies to advance medicine. Great respect is due for those who do these trials. However, limitations that might not be evident from a meta-analysis are worth noting. As seen in **Table 6**,[37–41] methods used to identify patients with delirium in some studies were not optimal.[37,42] In other studies, subtle baseline differences[40] and higher than expected rates of delirium[37,39] among the placebo group can make the intervention appear superior.

In summary, there are insufficient DB-RPCTs to recommend the use of any particular medication to either prevent or manage ("treat") delirium. Compared with nonpharmacologic interventions (see discussion in next section), pharmacologic interventions are less promising. Consistent with this, there are currently no US Food and Drug Administration–approved medications for delirium.

Table 4
Number of published double-blind, randomized placebo controlled trials for various pharmacologic agents for prevention and treatment of delirium based on category of patient populations

Pharmacologic Agent	Perioperative		ICU		Medical (Non-ICU)		Psychiatric Consultation		Palliative Care	
	Prev	Rx	Prev	Rx	Prev	Rx	Prev	Rx	Prev	Rx
Antipsychotics	6	1	1[a]	2	0	1	0	0	0	0
Melatonin agonist	2	0	0	0	2	0	0	0	0	0
Cholinesterase inhibitors	4	0	2[b]	0	0	0	0	0	0	0

Abbreviations: Prev, preventive studies; Rx, treatment studies.
[a] This study by Page et al, 2013, included both prevalent and incident cases of delirium.
[b] Although both studies in ICU, one study had 100% surgical patients; the other study had 69% surgical patients.

Table 5
Critical analysis of 3 frequently cited double-blind, randomized placebo-controlled intensive care unit studies of antipsychotics on prevention (Page) and treatment (Devlin, Girard) of delirium

Author, Year, Location	Sample Size		Age		Percent Intubated		Percent Medical		Intervention[a]	Primary Outcome and Results	Results		P Value	Bias Ratings[b]
	Int	Cntl	Int	Cntl	Int	Cntl	Int	Cntl			Int	Cntl		
Page et al,[34] 2013, UK	71	70	68	69	100	100	59	70	Haloperidol	Median number of days alive, delirium-free, and coma-free in first 14 d	5	6	.53	6
Girard et al,[36] 2010, US	30 36	35	54 56	51	100	100	57 67	64	Haloperidol or Ziprasodone	Median number of days alive, delirium-free and coma-free in first 21 d	14 15	12.5	.66	5
Devlin et al,[35] 2010, US	18	18	62	64	72	89	72	76	Quetiapine	Mean number of hours in delirium	36	120	.006	4

Limitations important for clinicians caring for older patients: Mean or median ages are lower than typical geriatric patients. Doses and frequency of antipsychotic medications used are higher than guidelines would recommend for older patients. Page and Girard studies excluded patients with moderate to severe dementia. Not noted in Devlin study.

General limitations to be aware of related to ICU delirium studies and meta-analyses that use these studies: These are very complex and difficult studies to perform because of the necessity of sedation, pain control, and additional antipsychotics in patients who are intubated. All 3 studies controlled for these variables. In the Page and Devlin studies, there were differences in amount of sedation medications. Both of these studies' authors suggest that the antipsychotic might reduce the need for sedatives. However, it is also possible that sedatives and opioids might be causing some delirium d/h in the placebo group. Could the benefit of antipsychotics be related to sedation rather than treating the underlying neurotransmitter mechanisms of delirium? Page study: Trend toward less sedation (total daily dose) for haloperidol group compared with placebo for opiates ($P = .06$ for fentanyl, $P = .23$ for morphine), propofol ($P = .06$). Additional open-label antipsychotic use: haloperidol group 8 (11%); placebo group 18 (26%); RR 0.44 (0.20–0.94). Devlin study: Before randomization, midazolam equivalents and haloperidol doses were the same, but there seemed to be large differences in fentanyl doses (Int = 0 [0–200] μg versus Cntl = 520 [0–1200] μg). (Authors did not report P values for this.) After randomization, there was a nonsignificant difference in midazolam equivalents (Int = 5.3 mg/d vs Cntl = 26.5 mg/d) and significantly higher fentanyl doses (Int = 0 [0–65] μg versus Cntl = 170 [14–1089] μg, $P = .02$). Girard study: All groups received similar doses per day of benzodiazepines ($P = .10$), opiates ($P = .87$), and propofol ($P = .16$). Additional haloperidol use was similar among all 3 groups: Average daily dose = 4.5 mg/5.7 mg/5.0 mg (haloperidol/ziprasodone/placebo groups), $P = .65$.

Abbreviations: Cntl, control; Int, intervention.

[a] Page: 2.5 mg IV every 8 hours; Girard: Haloperidol (5 mg/5 mL) or Ziprasodone a 40 mg/5 mL). Initiated every 12 h and then every 6 h for up to 14 d; Devlin: Initial dose 50 mg every 12 h, titrated upwards on a daily basis by increments of 50 mg every 12 h to a maximum dose of 200 mg every 12 h if the subject received at least one dose of as-needed haloperidol in the previous 24 h. All studies had matching placebo solutions.

[b] Risk of bias: uses ratings based on a 6-point scale, 1 point for each of the following areas: balance allocation, allocation concealment, blinding, outcome completion, outcome reporting complete, other bias. Higher score indicates less bias.

Table 6
Critical analysis of 6 frequently cited double-blind, randomized placebo controlled trials of antipsychotics related to peri-operative delirium

Author, Year, Location	Sample Size	Age	Type of Surgery	Intervention	Delirium Incidence (%)	P Value+	Bias Ratings[a]
Hakim et al,[37] 2012, Egypt	51 50	All >65	CABG or CABG with Valve	Risperidone 0.5 mg po every 12 h until ICSD = 0	7/51 (14%) 17/50 (34%)	.031	6
All patients had subsyndromal delirium (SSD, defined as ICDSC score 1–3). For delirium incidence, ICDSC used for identifying patients with possible delirium. Only patients with scores >4 were seen by a psychiatrist to confirm diagnosis of delirium. It is not clear what happened to the patients who did not increase their ICDSC >4. Did some of these have delirium not identified by the ICDSC? Furthermore, screening for delirium was not performed by research personnel but by different clinicians. Four intensivists and 3 ward physicians, trained in the use of ICDSC and blinded to the patients' groups, did the screening. Placebo group might be slightly higher than expected. In the authors' institution, previous data suggested that about 26% of patients with SSD, as they defined it, go onto delirium.							
Kalisvaart et al,[38] 2005, The Netherlands	212 218 80 80		Hip (~2/3 elective)	Haloperidol 0.5 mg po TID preop and postop days 1–3	32/212 (15%) 36/218 (17%)	NS	5
This study did not show difference in incidence. However, the haloperidol group had shorter duration of delirium. Larger standard deviation of severity score in placebo group compared with intervention group suggests outliers, which may have skewed results concerning duration of delirium. Subjects who dropped out of the study (~11%) were not included in final analysis.							
Wang et al,[41] 2012, China	229 228 74 74		Intra-abdominal (>70%), intrathoracic (11%–14%)	Haloperidol 0.5 mg IV bolus then 0.1 mg/h for 12 h[b]	35/229 (15%) 53/228 (23%)	.031	4
Incidence of delirium in the placebo group might be higher than expected, whereas the haloperidol group rates similar to observational studies. Study by Raats and colleagues[80] (78% colorectal, 22% abdominal aorta) had a rate of 15%. This study is sometimes used in meta-analyses or analyzed as an ICU study. It should not be. Average stay in ICU <24 h.							
Kaneko et al,[42] 1999, Japan	38 40 72 73		Elective gastrointestinal (gastrectomy, colectomy)	Haloperidol 5 mg IV every night postop days 1–5	4/38 (11%) 13/40 (33%)	<.05	3

Diagnosis of delirium was made retrospectively: "on the 5th day after surgery, postoperative data were collected from the patients and their nursing charts regarding (i) cognition, with particular attention to signs and symptoms of delirium, (ii) use of pain medication and (iii) sleep pattern, with special attention being paid to the sleep wakefulness rhythm. Psychotic diagnoses were based on the DSM-III-R." There was no mention of who did the data collection and if this/these person(s) were blinded.

Larsen et al,[39] 2010, US	196	204	73	74	Elective hip and knee replacement	Olanzapine 5 mg po once preop and postop day 1	28/196 (14%)	82/204 (40%)	<.0001	3

Placebo group had higher than expected rate of delirium (40%). No preoperative baseline mental status examination was performed. Seventeen more subjects in the control group (94/204) had ASA >3 compared with the intervention group (78/196). ASA status is a risk factor for postoperative delirium. Seemingly one of the best placebo RCTs in literature (especially because of large sample size), but impact factor of journal was 2.06 in year of publication, 2010.

Prakanrattana & Prapaitrakool,[40] 2007, Thailand	63	63	61	61	Cardiopulmonary bypass (~70% CABG, ~30% Valve)	Risperidone 1 mg[c]	7/63 (11%)	20/63 (32%)	.0009	3

Difference in "time from opening eyes to following commands (minutes)" between risperidone group (65.2 + 51) and placebo group (80.2 + 83; $P = .814$). This reported P value seems inaccurate. This might have had an impact on the primary outcome because most delirious patients in the placebo group (15/20) had delirium postoperatively on the day of surgery (risperidone group had 3/7 with delirium on day of surgery). Were some of the patients in the placebo group already delirious? In their analysis of factors associated with postoperative delirium among all subjects, "time from opening eyes to following commands" was an independent risk factor for delirium. This might also be related to possible differences in amounts of sedation and analgesia, which were not reported. The authors only describe the general techniques, medications, and ranges of usual doses for preoperative preparation (midazolam) and induction (thiopentene, midazolam, and fentanyl). This study is sometimes used in meta-analyses or analyzed as an ICU study. Although average stay in ICU was 3 d, it should be considered a postoperative delirium study.

Abbreviations: CABG, coronary artery bypass graft; ICDSC, Intensive Care Delirium Screening Checklist; po, orally; TID, 3 times a day.

[a] Risk of bias ratings based on a 6-point scale, 1 point for each of the following areas: balance allocation, allocation concealment, blinding, outcome completion, outcome reporting complete, other bias. Higher score indicates less bias.

[b] Started within 1 h of enrollment postoperatively.

[c] Started postoperatively when patient started waking up in the ICU; used disintegrating tablet; placebo was a Listerine antiseptic strip.

NONPHARMACOLOGIC PREVENTION AND TREATMENT

Although studies of pharmacologic treatment of delirium have limitations, there is a better developed and summarized literature on the use of multicomponent nonpharmacologic delirium prevention programs[32] that highlight that these programs carry more benefits than risk. Because the multicomponent strategies are complex, implementing within a health care system should be a strategic process (see **Box 4**).

Educational Programs

Frontline health care staff has a difficult time differentiating delirium and dementia.[43] Studies on educational/reorganization of nursing to assess and prevent delirium have demonstrated positive results in reducing incidence of delirium.[44–46] Although the item of the educational program in each study varied, they usually have bedside training and continuous support and emphasize a change in protocol or practice. The educational program is usually an integral part of the multicomponent strategies for delirium, so the effect of educational interventions itself cannot be assessed separately.

Multicomponent Nonpharmacologic Prevention

Because delirium develops based on several precipitating factors, a useful practical approach to prevent delirium has been to identify patients at risk for delirium and direct preventative strategies that target specific risk factors (**Table 7**). A recent systematic review[47] pooled the result of 11 multicomponent nonpharmacologic prevention studies and demonstrated significant reductions in delirium incidence (odds ratio [OR] 0.47, 95% confidence interval [CI] 0.38–0.58) and rate of falls (OR 0.38, 95% CI 0.25–0.60). Another systematic review[32] of 7 RCTs showed a reduction in the incidence of delirium compared with usual care in both medical (relative risk [RR] 0.63, 95% CI 0.43–0.92) and surgical wards (RR 0.71, 95% CI 0.59–0.85).

One of the well-known multicomponent nonpharmacologic models is the Hospital Elder Life Program (HELP) (http://www.hospitalelderlifeprogram.org). HELP is a patient-centered, multidisciplinary, and integrated model of care that uses multicomponent strategies for preventing delirium and functional decline in hospitalized older persons. The effectiveness of HELP for prevention of adverse hospital outcomes, including incident delirium,[48] cognitive and functional decline,[49] and hospital falls,[50,51] is well documented. HELP programs, based on volunteer effort, require significant infrastructure investments from the health care system.

Single Component Nonpharmacologic Prevention

Some examples of single component prevention studies include

- Music therapy (may lower the incidence of delirium compared with usual care but invalidated method of assessing delirium was used)[52,53]
- Dynamic light application in ICU (RCT: No effect; OR 1.24, 95% CI 0.92–1.68).[54]
- Care at home for older patients for some acute illnesses instead of traditional hospitalization (lower incidence of delirium and greater patient satisfaction compared with usual care in the hospital setting).[55,56]

Prevention of Delirium in Older People in Institutional Long-Term Care

Two studies were identified by a Cochrane Review,[57] both cluster RCTs. One (n = 3538, moderate-quality evidence) used a computerized system to identify deliriogenic medications, which led to a pharmacist-led medication review. Delirium incidence was decreased (12-month hazard ratio 0.42, CI 0.34–0.51), but there was no

Table 7
Mnemonic for identification of patients at risk for delirium and prevention strategies based on principles found in multicomponent prevention studies

	Risk Factors		Prevention Strategies
B	Baseline dementia?	P	Protocol for sleep (nonpharmacologic)
E	Eye problems?	R	Replenish fluids/recognize volume depletion
A	Altered sleep/wake cycle?	E	Ear aids (amplifiers, patient's hearing aids)
W	Water or dehydration problems?	V	Visual aids
A	Adding >3 medications, especially sedative/hypnotics?	E	Early ambulation
R	Restricted mobility?	N	Name person, place, time for reorientation
E	Ear problems?	T	Taper or discontinue unnecessary medications

reduction in hospital admissions, mortality, or falls risk. The other (n = 98) used a hydration-based intervention. There was no reduction in delirium incidence.

Nonpharmacologic Treatment

Nonpharmacologic approaches have been recommended as the first-line treatment of delirium, involving removal of the causes or exacerbating factors (eg, restraints, indwelling urinary catheters, unnecessary tubing, or telemetry), symptom management, and education of patient and family member or caregivers. Four RCTs[58–61] evaluated the role of comprehensive geriatric assessment and multicomponent nonpharmacologic strategies to manage delirium targeted at risk factors of delirium among elderly patients. Nonpharmacologic treatment approaches focused on consultation by geriatrician or psychiatrist and follow-up by a liaison nurse, orientation, therapeutic activities/cognitive stimulation, provision of familiar items and family presence, optimizing sensory input, avoidance of restraints, early mobilization, nutritional supplements, and comprehensive discharge planning. Two of the RCTs reported higher rates of recovery from delirium in the intervention group,[59,60] but did not decrease mortality and had no significant effect on length of hospital stay. Other non-RCTs showed that nonpharmacologic treatment had benefit in at least one of following outcomes: delirium duration, cognitive or physical function, length of stay, or costs.[45,62–64] A recent clinical practice guideline on the management of delirium recommends a multicomponent intervention.[9]

An alternative to these consultative models and an example of an implementation model was the establishment of a designated room for patients with delirium, called the delirium room (DR),[65] sometimes referred to as the delirium intensive care unit.[66] The DR is a 4-bed patient room within an acute care of the elderly unit that provides 24-hour nursing care and does not use physical restraints. The DR was developed based on the goal that delirium could be managed safely and effectively without the use of physical restraints by providing constant nurse supervision instead of 1:1 staff assignments. The DR demonstrated a significant effect for improving function among delirious patients[67] and has resulted in an educational and management tool called the T-A-DA method (Tolerate, Anticipate, Don't Agitate; https://www.youtube.com/watch?v=D70oGWJqPkl&feature=youtu.be).

Other studies have reported similar specialized medical hospital units for older adults with delirium showing promising results, including a trend toward lower mortality compared with usual care.[68–70] The benefits of implementing a designated location for patients with delirium include more focused and hands-on training of staff, increased awareness of delirium, and easier implementation of delirium interventions (eg, avoiding restraints, encouraging mobilization).

Another example of an implementation model used a process improvement strategy to improve use of the patient observers (1:1 caregivers) in a surgical trauma unit. Patients with delirium were identified as the most prevalent and concerning patient group. Patient observer direct-care hours decreased (median 208 h/wk to 112 h/wk); fall rate remained unchanged, while staff satisfaction increased from 9% to 72% and costs associated with providing observer care remained stable.[71]

THE FUTURE OF DELIRIUM

Delirium is gaining increased recognition as a scientific discipline. There are now professional societies representing America, Australasia, and Europe.[72] A federation of these societies (iDelirium.org) has been working together to educate a broader audience, collaborate on research, and raise awareness as a unified body for delirium advancement. As an example, members of these associations recently developed a consensus paper on the diagnosis of delirium superimposed on dementia and have plans for systematically examining biomarkers of delirium including electroencephalogram, imaging, and laboratory tests.

SUMMARY

Delirium is characterized by an acute change in attention and awareness that affects all cognitive processing. Despite the seriousness of the consequences of delirium and the availability of screening tools, it is often ignored by the health care system. Although rapid screening tools are available, clinicians caring for older patients need to have a good understanding of how to recognize and diagnose delirium even when confounding factors such as dementia are present. Patients with delirium may present differently depending on the setting, and different phenotypes are being recognized as the field evolves. Even the best studies of antipsychotics for delirium have limitations: most focus on perioperative and ICU populations, and results do not support the use of antipsychotics for delirium. Nonpharmacologic delirium prevention and management models exist, and strategies for the implementation of these programs are as important as the models themselves.

REFERENCES

1. Meagher DJ, Morandi A, Inouye SK, et al. Concordance between DSM-IV and DSM-5 criteria for delirium diagnosis in a pooled database of 768 prospectively evaluated patients using the delirium rating scale-revised-98. BMC Med 2014; 12:164–8.
2. European Delirium Association, American Delirium Society. The DSM-5 criteria, level of arousal and delirium diagnosis: inclusiveness is safer. BMC Med 2014; 12:141.
3. Lipowski ZJ. Delirium: acute brain failure in man. Springfield (IL): Thomas; 1980.
4. Pandharipande PP, Girard TD, Jackson JC, et al. Long-term cognitive impairment after critical illness. N Engl J Med 2013;369:1306–16.
5. Inouye SK, Kosar CM, Tommet D, et al. The CAM-S: development and validation of a new scoring system for delirium severity in 2 cohorts. Ann Intern Med 2014; 160:526–33.
6. Han JH, Zimmerman EE, Cutler N, et al. Delirium in older emergency department patients: recognition, risk factors, and psychomotor subtypes. Acad Emerg Med 2009;16:193–200.
7. Rice KL, Bennett MJ, Clesi T, et al. Mixed-methods approach to understanding nurses' clinical reasoning in recognizing delirium in hospitalized older adults. J Contin Educ Nurs 2014;45:136–48.
8. Clegg A, Westby M, Young JB. Under-reporting of delirium in the NHS. Age Ageing 2011;40:283–6.
9. DELIRIUM: diagnosis, prevention and management clinical guideline 103. Regent's Park, London: National Clinical Guideline Centre; 2010.
10. NIH REPORT: Research Program Online Reporting Tool. National Institutes of Health; 2016. Available at: http://projectreporter.nih.gov/reporter.cfm. Accessed August 9, 2016.
11. Posner MI, Petersen SE. The attention system of the human brain. Annu Rev Neurosci 1990;13:25–42.
12. Petersen SE, Posner MI. The attention system of the human brain: 20 years after. Annu Rev Neurosci 2012;35:73–89.

13. Cordell CB, Borson S, Boustani M. Alzheimer's Association recommendations for operationalizing the detection of cognitive impairment during the Medicare annual wellness visit in a primary care setting. Alzheimers Dement 2013;9: 141–50.

14. Leonard M, Adamis D, Saunders J, et al. A longitudinal study of delirium phenomenology indicates widespread neural dysfunction. Palliat Support Care 2015;13: 187–96.

15. American Psychiatric Association. Diagnostic and Statistical Manual of Mental Disorders. 5th edition. Washington, DC: American Psychiatric Association; 2013.

16. Inouye SK, Robinson T, Blaum C, et al. Postoperative delirium in older adults: best practice statement from the american geriatrics society. J Am Coll Surg 2014;272: 136–48.

17. Wei LA, Fearing MA, Sternberg EJ, et al. The confusion assessment method: a systematic review of current usage. J Am Coll Surg 2008;56:823–30.

18. Inouye SK, Foreman MD, Mion LC, et al. Nurses' recognition of delirium and its symptoms: comparison of nurse and researcher ratings. Arch Intern Med 2001; 161:2467–73.

19. Gaudreau JD, Gagnon P, Harel F, et al. Fast, systematic, and continuous delirium assessment in hospitalized patients: the nursing delirium screening scale. J Pain Symptom Manage 2005;29:368–75.

20. Koster S, Hensens AG, Oosterveld FG, et al. The delirium observation screening scale recognizes delirium early after cardiac surgery. Eur J Cardiovasc Nurs 2009;8:309–14.

21. Voyer P, Champoux N, Desrosiers J, et al. Recognizing acute delirium as part of your routine [RADAR]: a validation study. BMC Nurs 2015;14:19.

22. Bellelli G, Morandi A, Davis DH, et al. Validation of the 4AT, a new instrument for rapid delirium screening: a study in 234 hospitalised older people. Age Ageing 2014;43:496–502.

23. Damschroder LJ, Aron DC, Keith RE, et al. Fostering implementation of health services research findings into practice: a consolidated framework for advancing implementation science. Implement Sci 2009;4:1035–9.

24. Lin JS. Brain structure and mechanisms involved in the control of cortical activation and wakefulness, with emphasis on the posterior hypothalamus and histaminergic neurons. Sleep Med Rev 2000;4:471–503.

25. Giacino JT, Fins JJ, Laureys S, et al. Disorders of consciousness after acquired brain injury: the state of the science. Nat Rev Neurol 2014;10:99–114.

26. Tieges Z, Aisling M, Hall HR, et al. Abnormal level of arousal as a predictor of delirium and inattention: an exploratory study. Am J Geriatr Psychiatry 2013;21: 1244–53.

27. Chester JG, Beth Harrington M, Rudolph JL. Serial administration of a modified Richmond agitation and sedation scale for delirium screening. J Hosp Med 2012;7:450–3.

28. Yevchak AM, Doherty K, Kelly B, et al. The association between an ultrabrief cognitive screening in older adults and hospital outcomes. J Hosp Med 2015; 10:651–7.

29. Yevchak AM, Jin HH, Doherty K, et al. Impaired arousal in older adults is associated with prolonged hospital stay and discharge to skilled nursing facility. J Am Med Dir Assoc 2015;16:586–9.

30. Maldonado JR. Neuropathogenesis of delirium: review of current etiologic theories and common pathways. Am J Geriatr Psychiatry 2013;21:1190–222.

31. Neufeld KJ, Yue J, Robinson TN, et al. Antipsychotic medication for prevention and treatment of delirium in hospitalized adults: a systematic review and meta-analysis. J Am Geriatr Soc 2016;64:705–14.

32. Siddiqi N, Harrison JK, Clegg A, et al. Interventions for preventing delirium in hospitalised non-ICU patients. Cochrane Database Syst Rev 2016;3:CD005563.

33. Al-Qadheeb NS, Balk EM, Fraser GL, et al. Randomized ICU trials do not demonstrate an association between interventions that reduce delirium duration and short-term mortality: a systematic review and meta-analysis. Crit Care Med 2014;42:1442–54.

34. Page VJ, Ely EW, Gates S, et al. Effect of intravenous haloperidol on the duration of delirium and coma in critically ill patients (Hope-ICU): a randomised, double-blind, placebo-controlled trial. Lancet Respir Med 2013;1:515–23.

35. Devlin JW, Roberts RJ, Fong JJ, et al. Efficacy and safety of quetiapine in critically ill patients with delirium: a prospective, multicenter, randomized, double-blind, placebo-controlled pilot study. Crit Care Med 2010;38:419–27.

36. Girard TD, Pandharipande PP, Carson SS, et al. Feasibility, efficacy, and safety of antipsychotics for intensive care unit delirium: the MIND randomized, placebo-controlled trial. Crit Care Med 2010;38:428–37.

37. Hakim SM, Othman AI, Naoum DO. Early treatment with risperidone for subsyndromal delirium after on-pump cardiac surgery in the elderly: a randomized trial. Anesthesiology 2012;116:987–97.

38. Kalisvaart KJ, de Jonghe JF, Bogaards MJ, et al. Haloperidol prophylaxis for elderly hip-surgery patients at risk for delirium: a randomized placebo-controlled study. J Am Geriatr Soc 2005;53:1658–66.

39. Larsen KA, Kelly SE, Stern TA, et al. Administration of olanzapine to prevent postoperative delirium in elderly joint-replacement patients: a randomized, controlled trial. Psychosomatics 2010;51:409–18.

40. Prakanrattana U, Prapaitrakool S. Efficacy of risperidone for prevention of postoperative delirium in cardiac surgery. Anaesth Intensive Care 2007;35:714–9.

41. Wang W, Li HL, Wang DX, et al. Haloperidol prophylaxis decreases delirium incidence in elderly patients after noncardiac surgery: a randomized controlled trial*. Crit Care Med 2012;40:731–9.

42. Kaneko T, Cai J, Ishikura T, et al. Prophylactic consecutive administration of haloperidol can reduce the occurrence of postoperative delirium in gastrointestinal surgery. Yonago Acta Med 1999;42:179–84.

43. Steis MR, Fick DM. Delirium superimposed on dementia: accuracy of nurse documentation. J Gerontol Nurs 2012;38:32–42.

44. Lundstrom M, Edlund A, Karlsson S, et al. A multifactorial intervention program reduces the duration of delirium, length of hospitalization, and mortality in delirious patients. J Am Geriatr Soc 2005;53:622–8.

45. Milisen K, Foreman MD, Abraham IL, et al. A nurse-led interdisciplinary intervention program for delirium in elderly hip-fracture patients. J Am Geriatr Soc 2001; 49:523–32.

46. Tabet N, Hudson S, Sweeney V, et al. An educational intervention can prevent delirium on acute medical wards. Age Ageing 2005;34:152–6.

47. Hshieh TT, Yue J, Oh E, et al. Effectiveness of multicomponent nonpharmacological delirium interventions: a meta-analysis. JAMA Intern Med 2015;175:512–20.

48. Inouye SK, Bogardus ST Jr, Charpentier PA, et al. A multicomponent intervention to prevent delirium in hospitalized older patients. N Engl J Med 1999;340:669–76.

49. Inouye SK, Bogardus ST Jr, Baker DI, et al. The hospital elder life program: a model of care to prevent cognitive and functional decline in older hospitalized patients. Hospital elder life program. J Am Geriatr Soc 2000;48:1697–706.

50. Caplan G, Harper E. Recruitment of volunteers to improve vitality in the elderly: the REVIVE study. Intern Med J 2007;37:95–100.

51. Inouye SK, Brown CJ, Tinetti ME. Medicare nonpayment, hospital falls, and unintended consequences. N Engl J Med 2009;360:2390–3.

52. McCaffrey R, Locsin R. The effect of music listening on acute confusion and delirium in elders undergoing elective hip and knee surgery. J Clin Nurs 2004; 13:91–6.

53. McCaffrey R, Locsin R. The effect of music on pain and acute confusion in older adults undergoing hip and knee surgery. Holist Nurs Pract 2006;20:218–24 [quiz: 25–6].

54. Simons KS, Laheij RJ, van den Boogaard M, et al. Dynamic light application therapy to reduce the incidence and duration of delirium in intensive-care patients: a randomised controlled trial. Lancet Respir Med 2016;4:194–202.

55. Caplan GA, Ward JA, Brennan NJ, et al. Hospital in the home: a randomised controlled trial. Med J Aust 1999;170:156–60.

56. Caplan GA, Coconis J, Board N, et al. Does home treatment affect delirium? A randomised controlled trial of rehabilitation of elderly and care at home or usual treatment (The REACH-OUT trial). Age Ageing 2006;35:53–60.

57. Clegg A, Siddiqi N, Holt R, et al. Interventions for preventing delirium in older people in institutional long term care. Cochrane Database Syst Rev 2014;(1):CD009537.

58. Cole MG, Primeau FJ, Bailey RF, et al. Systematic intervention for elderly inpatients with delirium: a randomized trial. CMAJ 1994;151:965–70.

59. Cole MG, McCusker J, Bellavance F, et al. Systematic detection and multidisciplinary care of delirium in older medical inpatients: a randomized trial. CMAJ 2002;167:753–9.

60. Pitkala KH, Laurila JV, Strandberg TE, et al. Multicomponent geriatric intervention for elderly inpatients with delirium: a randomized, controlled trial. J Gerontol A Biol Sci Med Sci 2006;61:176–81.

61. Mador JE, Giles L, Whitehead C, et al. A randomized controlled trial of a behavior advisory service for hospitalized older patients with confusion. Int J Geriatr Psychiatry 2004;19:858–63.

62. Rubin FH, Neal K, Fenlon K, et al. Sustainability and scalability of the hospital elder life program at a community hospital. J Am Coll Surg 2011;59:359–65.

63. Zaubler TS, Murphy K, Rizzuto L, et al. Quality improvement and cost savings with multicomponent delirium interventions: replication of the hospital elder life program in a community hospital. Psychosomatics 2013;54:219–26.

64. Chen CC, Lin MT, Tien YW, et al. Modified hospital elder life program: effects on abdominal surgery patients. J Am Coll Surg 2011;213:245–52.

65. Flaherty JH, Tariq SH, Raghavan S, et al. A model for managing delirious older inpatients. J Am Geriatr Soc 2003;51:1031–5.

66. Flaherty JH, Morley JE. Delirium in the nursing home. J Am Med Dir Assoc 2013; 14:632–4.

67. Flaherty JH, Steele DK, Chibnall JT, et al. An ACE unit with a delirium room may improve function and equalize length of stay among older delirious medical inpatients. J Gerontol A Biol Sci Med Sci 2010;65:1387–92.

68. Mudge AM, Maussen C, Duncan J, et al. Improving quality of delirium care in a general medical service with established interdisciplinary care: a controlled trial. Intern Med J 2013;43:270–7.
69. Eeles E, Thompson L, McCrow J, et al. Management of delirium in medicine: experience of a close observation unit. Australas J Ageing 2013;32:60–3.
70. Wong Tin Niam DM, Geddes JA, Inderjeeth CA. Delirium unit: our experience. Australas J Ageing 2009;28:206–10.
71. Rachh P, Wilkins G, Capodilupo TA, et al. Redesigning the patient observer model to achieve increased efficiency and staff engagement on a surgical trauma inpatient unit. Jt Comm J Qual Patient Saf 2016;42:77–87.
72. Rudolph JL, Boustani M, Kamholz B, et al. Delirium: a strategic plan to bring an ancient disease into the 21st century. J Am Coll Surg 2011;59(Suppl 2):S237–40.
73. Inouye SK, Westendorp RG, Saczynski JS. Delirium in elderly people. Lancet 2014;383:911–22.
74. Ljubisavljevic V, Kelly B. Risk factors for development of delirium among oncology patients. Gen Hosp Psychiatry 2003;25:345–52.
75. Centeno C, Sanz A, Bruera E. Delirium in advanced cancer patients. Palliat Med 2004;18:184–94.
76. Breitbart W, Strout D. Delirium in the terminally ill. Clin Geriatr Med 2000;16:357–72.
77. Casarett DJ, Inouye SK. Diagnosis and management of delirium near the end of life. Ann Intern Med 2001;135:32–40.
78. Barron EA, Holmes J. Delirium within the emergency care setting, occurrence and detection: a systematic review. Emerg Med J 2013;30:263–8.
79. Pitkala KH, Laurila JV, Strandberg TE, et al. Prognostic significance of delirium in frail older people. Dement Geriatr Cogn Disord 2005;19:158–63.
80. Raats JW, van Eijsden WA, Crolla RM, et al. Risk factors and outcomes for post-operative delirium after major surgery in elderly patients. PLos One 2015;10:e0136071.

Integrating Quality Palliative and End-of-Life Care into the Geriatric Assessment

Opportunities and Challenges

Daniel Swagerty, MD, MPH

KEYWORDS

- Palliative care • End-of-life care • Prognosis • Disease trajectories
- Symptom management

KEY POINTS

- The comprehensive geriatric assessment is greatly enhanced by integration of ongoing palliative and end-of-life care assessments and care.
- Advance care planning and discussions about advanced illness management and dying can improve end-of-life care outcomes.
- Common disease trajectories are evident that indicate a limited life expectancy and the need for palliative care.
- Common physiologic and physical changes are evident, which can be used to improve palliative and end-of-life symptom management.
- Anticipation and management of the common physical, psychosocial, and spiritual symptoms experienced at the end of life are vital to a quality death for older adults.

INTRODUCTION

Traditionally, health care providers have had difficulty discussing nonaggressive options of care with their patients because it is often associated with giving up. In particular, physicians may believe in the value of palliative care but still hesitate to bring up the subject with their patients, fearing that it will destroy their hope or imply a lack of commitment to treatment.[1,2] This circumstance commonly results in unnecessary, nontherapeutic, expensive treatments and decreased quality of life.[3] It is imperative that the ongoing assessment of older adults includes the appropriate and timely consideration, then completion, of transitioning from conventional curative care treatments to a palliative or comfort care model of care. These care transitions should

Department of Family Medicine, Landon Center on Aging, University of Kansas School of Medicine, 3901 Rainbow Boulevard, Kansas City, KS, USA
E-mail address: dswagert@kumc.edu

Clin Geriatr Med 33 (2017) 415–429
http://dx.doi.org/10.1016/j.cger.2017.03.005
0749-0690/17/© 2017 Elsevier Inc. All rights reserved.

geriatric.theclinics.com

focus on improving quality of life through shared decision-making between patients, their families when appropriate, and health care providers.[4] In general, there needs to be greater recognition and implementation of palliative care to improve older adult patients' quality of life and their deaths through symptom control and follow-through on their health care choices.

Palliative care is frequently perceived as an end-of-life measure, an option only when curative or life-prolonging therapy is no longer beneficial. This perception is false in that palliative care, including symptom management, psychosocial counseling, and discussion about treatment goals and expectations, should be incorporated into the routine assessment and primary care of older adults beginning at the time of any new diagnosis, particularly for patients with aggressive disease or high symptom burden. It can be the main focus of care or offered concurrently with life-prolonging medical treatment.[5]

SCOPE AND DEFINITION OF PALLIATIVE AND END-OF-LIFE CARE

Palliative care, at its best, provides excellent symptom management and exceptional patient, family, intraprofessional, and interprofessional communication regarding illness, hopes, goals, and expectations for treatment over time, toward the goal of creating a patient-centered plan of care.[6] An interprofessional team care approach is optimal to achieve the aims of relieving suffering, improving the quality of life, optimizing function, and assisting with decision-making for patients with advanced illness and their families.[7,8] This approach is effective for providing comprehensive, proactive assessments and monitoring with advanced symptom management and counseling. Further, it allows for coordination with community services to furnish medical equipment, meals, transportation, caregiving, and other services needed to improve overall quality of life and wellness.

Through shared decision-making, older adult patients can receive relief of their physical and emotional suffering as well as preventing unnecessary hospitalizations, medications, and treatments. A primary goal for these patients is an improved quality of life, the highest practicable functional status, and greater satisfaction with their health care, while also reducing the total costs of care.[3]

The goals of palliative and end-of-life care are 4-fold: (1) advanced symptom management at home or the least restrictive environment, care coordination with community service providers, and an interprofessional approach to complex quality-of-life issues; (2) facilitated shared decision-making by and between the patients, their families when appropriate, and their physician through development of innovative standardized tools for each party; (3) quality-of-life focused treatment choices with a decrease or elimination of multiple inpatient and outpatient services; and (4) a seamless continuum of community-based supportive care until the end of life. Palliative care is best offered in the last 2 years of life, if not initially from the time of any new life-limiting diagnosis. End-of-life care aims to relieve suffering and improve quality of life for patients with advanced illness and their families in the last days of life.[7,8]

Providing outstanding palliative and end-of-life care is not merely practical but imperative for older adult patients. It enhances quality of care when added to the work done by the health care team caring for older adults. The successful integration of palliative care into routine geriatric assessment should result in fewer deaths in a hospital setting, longer hospice lengths of stay, less futile treatments in the last weeks of life, and higher satisfaction levels for patients and families.

QUALITY OF DEATH

The deaths of older adults in developed countries worldwide are typically slow and associated with chronic disease in persons with multiple problems. These deaths are usually notable for a marked increase in dependency and care needs. The quality of life experienced by these dying older adults is often poor because of inadequate treatment of distress and symptoms, fragmented care, as well as strains on the family and support system. Difficult decisions about the use of life-prolonging treatments are also commonly necessary but not always addressed.[9] **Box 1** provides an overview of the advantages of palliative and end-of-life care for the terminally ill. The health care team caring for older adults should strive to incorporate a palliative care approach into their ongoing routine and periodic comprehensive assessment of their patients to provide those with life-limiting and threatening illness the greatest benefit toward their quality of life and function.[10]

PROGNOSTICATION

It is important to convey the prognosis as accurate as possible to patients as they tend to have an optimism bias toward the life-extending benefit of palliative care.[11–13] Similarly, physicians tend to be overly optimistic in their prognosis. Their inaccuracies tend to be systematically optimistic and not restricted to certain types of physician or to certain types of patients.[14] An accurate prognosis is important for conveying accurate information in advance care planning and discussions about palliative care and dying as well as improving end-of-life care outcomes. In particular, poor prognostication can lead to underuse of palliative care and end-of-life care services, overuse of preventative screening and curative care treatments, as well as a delay in advance care planning and conversations about death and dying.[11]

Many physicians are uncomfortable with prognosticating, with studies showing their accuracy to be as poor as 20%.[14,15] Physician awareness of death trajectories can be helpful.[16] Historically, life expectancy was low and death rates high. The dying trajectory was short.[17] People were generally healthy until they became ill; then they died,

---

Box 1
Advantages of palliative and end-of-life care for the terminally ill

- Better pain and symptom assessment and management
- Lower rates of inappropriate medication usage
- Medical goal becomes pain relief and symptom control
- Less physical restraints, tube feedings, IVs, unwarranted therapies, hospitalizations, life-prolonging treatments
- Terminally ill residents kept in their own environment
- Health professional and interprofessional services provided beyond those usually offered
- Management of terminal patients' increasing hygienic needs
- Improved emotional and spiritual support
- End-of-life education and bereavement support for families and nursing staff
- Prolonged visits for compassionate listening and companionship
- Providing medications and medical supplies related to the terminal diagnosis
- Greater satisfaction of surviving families with the care provided to patients

mostly from infectious diseases. This dying trajectory is shown in **Fig. 1**. People did not live long enough to die of chronic diseases. Advances in public sanitation and medical science over the last 100 years has created chronic disease.[18] Before the twentieth century, very few curable diseases existed. The practice of medicine primarily involved palliating and alleviating symptoms, as described by an eighteenth century aphorism: *to cure sometimes, to relieve often, to comfort always*.[16] By the mid-twentieth century, clean water, improved nutrition, vaccine, antibiotics, anesthetics, and improved diagnostic techniques and surgical procedures had changed the death trajectory (see **Fig. 1**) from describing death from sudden disease to one from acute trauma. Currently, only 10% of people have this death trajectory.

Thus, the nature of medicine changed from palliation to cure in the twentieth century, as illustrated by the aphorism: *to comfort sometimes, to relieve often, to cure always*. Modern medicine has cured many of the causes of premature death, thus creating a death for most people to be from chronic disease. The twentieth century health care professional began to accept nothing short of cure, and the old dying trajectory changed. Dying became much more complex and of a much longer duration as shown in **Figs. 2** and **3**. Currently, 90% of people now live long enough to die of diseases, such as congestive heart disease, chronic obstructive pulmonary disease, cancers, renal failure, and dementia. Dying now occurs over an average of 30 months, with some diseases, such as Alzheimer disease, having a duration of dying of more than 10 years.[16] **Fig. 2** illustrates a death trajectory of progressive decline with episodic crises after a terminal diagnosis is established, as would be experienced by those with chronic heart, lung, and renal disease, as well as some cancers. This death trajectory is currently experienced by 60% of people, whereas 30% of people have a lingering, expected death trajectory as shown in (see **Fig. 3**). Some cancers and most dementias are characterized by this death trajectory.

Fortunately, modern medicine is beginning to recognize its limitations. Despite medical miracles, such as organ transplants and effective cancer treatments, everyone still eventually dies. We are now increasingly faced with considering what is best for patients and their families given the complexity of balancing the risk and benefits of modern health care screening, diagnostic assessments, and treatments. Consideration must now be given much more commonly to when the curative care approach should be stopped, a time beyond which we are causing more burden for our patients and their families by taking away their control, their dignity, and their finances.[16] There are tremendous physical, social, and economic implications of what we can offer through modern medical science. Our challenge is to more accurately prognosticate,

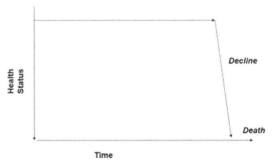

Fig. 1. Sudden illness/trauma without prior comorbidity.

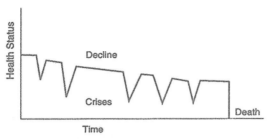

Fig. 2. Progressive decline with episodic crisis.

communicate, and educate so as to provide the excellent and timely palliative and end-of-life care that our patients deserve. Our twenty-first century aphorism should be *to cure when it is reasonable, to relieve symptoms often, to comfort always.*[16]

THE TRANSITION FROM CURATIVE TO PALLIATIVE CARE

Modern medicine is generally still in the cure mode, with every symptom and problem seen as a challenge to diagnosis and treat.[19] A cure is often the only goal we strive to meet, which often results in failure. Wise health care providers do not give up on their patients but recognize when to transition from diagnose and treat to palliate.[5] The curative care model, shown in **Fig. 4**, is one in which we seek to diagnose and treat every problem that arises.[20] All interventions are aimed at curative and life-prolonging measures, until it is abruptly realized that these curative measures have been unsuccessful. At that point, the focus may shift to symptom control and palliation. Death eventually occurs, with some providers still shocked and surprised.

An alternative trajectory to the curative care model is to include palliative care measures from the time of diagnosis of a life-limiting disease. In the palliative care model, shown in **Fig. 5**, supportive care and symptom control start early in the disease process.[20] Once a terminal diagnosis is established, a smooth transition from curative to palliative care measures can occur.[21] As the terminal phase progresses, there is more emphasis on palliation and less on curative and life-prolonging therapy. Once patients reach the end of their life, treatment is entirely palliation. When death occurs, no one is surprised because there has been an evolution in the care being provided. Patients, families, and health care providers are all much better prepared for the death. Families and health care providers are also better prepared for the subsequent bereavement.[19]

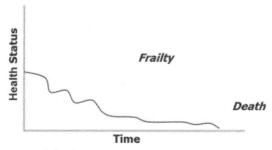

Fig. 3. Lingering, expected death.

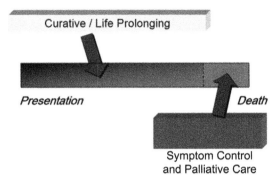

Fig. 4. Curative care model.

DETERMINING LIFE EXPECTANCY

Life expectancy can be difficult to determine during the course of a terminal illness. However, it is very common for individuals, and their families, at the end of their life to ask how long they have to live. It is best to answer this question in general rather than specific terms, using phases such as

- Months to years
- Weeks to months
- Days to weeks
- Hours to days

In considering life expectancy, providers should consider some of the common signs accompanying the dying process as shown in **Box 2**, with the caveat that every patient's death has its own individual process.[22] Sharing this information with patients and families can be extremely important in helping educate them about the dying process. It can also greatly assist them in accepting and acclimating to the progression of the terminal disease. Providers should never assume anyone knows anything about the natural dying process. In these circumstances, knowledge is power and one wants that power to reside as much as possible with patients and their families.

There are also several common prognostic indicators that are useful in considering life expectancy and communicating with patients and their families, as shown in **Box 3**. In addition, there are disease-specific prognostic guidelines for a variety of diseases. For example, a patient with AIDS being actively treated would have a poor prognosis when they have an elevated viral load, a dropping CD4 count (<50), a multiple drug–resistant virus, and are experiencing clinical deterioration. Similarly,

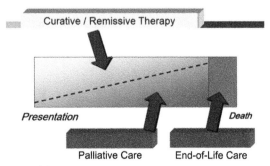

Fig. 5. Palliative care model.

Box 2
Common signs accompanying the dying process

Weeks to months

- Increased fatigue and sleep
- Decreased appetite, weight loss
- Talk about dying
- Increased discomfort
- Decreased ability to perform activities of daily living

Days to weeks

- Very poor appetite
- Nausea
- Rapid or labored respirations
- Excess pulmonary and/or gastric secretions
- Deceased alertness but responsive
- Decreased blood pressure
- Increased pulse
- Decreased urinary output

Hours to days

- No appetite
- Change in level of conscious
- Dreams or visions of deceased loved ones
- Disorientation
- Agitation
- Unable to follow simple commands
- Loss of gag reflex
- Picking at clothes or the air
- Unable to speak
- Unable to walk, if previously able
- Diaphoresis
- Poor thermoregulation
- Rapid pulse and respirations
- Decreased blood pressure
- Incontinence, if previously continent
- Bed bound

---

patients with end-stage chronic obstructive pulmonary disease should be recognized as having a poor prognosis in the presence of right heart failure, hypoxia at rest on supplemental oxygen, hypercapnia, unintentional progressive weight loss, and a resting tachycardia.

The best-known disease-specific prognostic indicators are those for determining eligibility of the US Medicare hospice benefit. The Centers for Medicare and Medicaid

---

Box 3
Common prognostic indicators

- Rapid progression of disease
- Significant functional decline
  ○ FAST, PPS, BADLs, NYHA
- Nutritional compromise
  ○ Weight loss of 5% in 1 month or 10% in 6 months
  ○ Serum albumin level less than 2.5 mg/dL
- Frequent emergency department/physician visits
- Two or more hospitalizations in 12 months for dehydration or advancement of the life-limiting disease
- Patients/families seeking care focused on comfort rather than cure

Abbreviations: BADLs, basic activities of daily living; FAST, Functional Assessment Staging Test; NYHA, New York Heart Association classification; PPS, Palliative Performance Scale.

---

established medical criteria for determining prognosis for cancer and noncancer diagnoses.[23] Patients with cancer who are determined to be hospice appropriate by their attending physician are not required to meet any other clinical guideline. All of these criteria were formulated under the auspices that they provide a reasonable estimate that patients' life expectancy is 6 months or less, with 2 physicians attesting to this prognosis, if the disease runs its normal course. Even if patients live longer than 6 months, eligibility can continue if (1) the prognosis remains 6 months or less, (2) the disease-specific guidelines continue to be met, and (3) patients demonstrate ongoing decline. These guidelines assume that the patients'/families' treatment goals are focused on symptom relief rather than the cure of underlying disease. The guidelines span cancer, dementia, human immunodeficiency virus/AIDS, as well as end-stage neurologic, pulmonary, cardiac, and renal disease. Perhaps best known to and used by both primary care and specialty physicians primarily caring for older adults are the guidelines for dementia, as shown in **Box 4**.

As is well known to those caring for older adults at the end of their lives, use of the Medicare hospice eligibility guidelines can present several challenges, with an accurate estimation of a 6-month or less life expectancy being chief among them. Prognosis is a major issue in qualifying many of our older adults for the hospice benefit for such reasons as

- Only some conditions have a clear prognosis of 6 months or less.
- There are not guidelines for all the pertinent diagnoses.
- Patients may not meet all guidelines for a condition, especially frail older adults.
- Significant comorbidities and the constellation of conditions matter a great deal in frail older adults.
- Current medical information/practices may not be reflected in the guidelines.
- Physicians are often too optimistic in prognoses.

In addressing some of the limitations of the disease-specific Medicare hospice eligibility guidelines, many providers have found the Palliative Performance Scale (PPS) to be a more useful tool in predicting poor survival. As shown in **Table 1**, the PPS score takes into account ambulation, activity, self-care, intake, and conscious level, all of which are much more patient centered than reliance on disease-specific criteria.[24] A PPS score of 50% or less generally indicates a prognosis of 6 months or less.

Box 4
Dementia

Criteria for eligibility for Medicare hospice benefit

- Stage 7 or beyond according to the FAST scale
- Unable to ambulate without assistance
- Unable to dress without assistance
- Unable to bathe without assistance
- Urinary or fecal incontinence, intermittent or constant
- No meaningful verbal communication, stereotypical phrases only, or ability to speak limited to 6 or fewer intelligible words
- Plus one of the following within the past 12 months
  - Aspiration pneumonia
  - Pyelonephritis or other upper urinary tract infection
  - Septicemia
  - Multiple stage 3 or 4 decubitus ulcers
  - Fever that recurs after antibiotic therapy
  - Inability to maintain sufficient fluid and calorie intake, with 10% weight loss during the previous 6 months or serum albumin level less than 2.5 g/dL (25 g/L)

PALLIATIVE CLINICAL CARE

Providing palliative clinical care, whether it is in the last few years or weeks of life, is much like providing good geriatric care to all older adults. One must consider the physiology changes in older adults such as homeo-stenosis of most (if not all) organ systems, changes in immunity, and changes in pharmacokinetics and pharmacodynamics. Thus, all treatment and medication use must take these considerations into account. Starting with the initial diagnosis of the life-limiting diagnosis, the provider must perform ongoing assessments for pain and nonpain symptoms, distress from any cause, concerns regarding decision-making, and assisting with advance care planning.[4,11] Some of the most common symptoms at the end of life are

- Anorexia/cachexia
- Anxiety
- Constipation
- Delirium
- Depression
- Dyspnea
- Drowsiness
- Fatigue
- Nausea/vomiting
- Secretions
- Pain

The provider should ask patients or family members about the severity of the symptom on a scale of 1 to 10, including the usual severity and how they would report the symptom at that time, how severe the symptom is at its best and its worst, and what level is tolerable for patients. Patients should also be asked how much the symptom impacts their daily life and how bothersome the symptom is to them.[11] This strategy will be important to continue for the duration of the life-limiting diagnosis, both in

Table 1
Palliative Performance Scale

%	Ambulation	Activity and Evidence of Disease	Self-Care	Intake	Conscious Level
100	Full	Normal activity, no evidence of disease	Full	Normal	Full
90	Full	Normal activity, some evidence of disease	Full	Normal	Full
80	Full	Normal activity with effort, some evidence of disease	Full	Normal or reduced	Full
70	Reduced	Unable normal job/work, some evidence of disease	Full	Normal or reduced	Full
60	Reduced	Unable hobby/house work, significant disease	Occasional assistance necessary	Normal or reduced	Full or confusion
50	Mainly Sit/Lie	Unable to do any work, extensive disease	Considerable assistance required	Normal or reduced	Full or confusion
40	Mainly in bed	Unable to do any work extensive disease	Mainly assistance	Normal or reduced	Full or drowsy or confusion
30	Totally bed bound	Unable to do any work, extensive disease	Total care	Reduced	Full or drowsy or confusion
20	Totally bed bound	Unable to do any work, extensive disease	Total care	Minimal sips	Full or drowsy or confusion
10	Totally bed bound	Unable to do any work, extensive disease	Total care	Mouth care only	Drowsy or coma

controlling the end-of-life symptoms and ongoing discussion of the goals of care. It is especially important as the disease progresses that patients, their families, and providers communicate about any change in advance directives and/or need to involve a surrogate decision maker.

CLINICAL CARE AT THE END OF LIFE

Using the same strategy since the life-limiting disease was diagnosed, the provider must perform ongoing assessments for the adequacy of symptom management as patients enter into the last few days of their life. The primary aim is to relieve suffering and any distress in an effort to provide the best possible quality of death for the patients and their families. However, it is not always apparent who is in the last 72 hours of their life. Even though we cannot always predict impending death, some things are fairly universal. The most common physical changes at the end of life are provided in **Boxes 5–7**. These changes in patients' central nervous, respiratory, circulatory, genitourinary, and gastrointestinal systems tend to be fairly consistent across patients as they enter into the last 72 hours of their life and are useful for planning changes in care, goals of care, and education of family and staff.

In the last few days of life, it is especially important to recognize and address the psychosocial needs of patients and their family members. There is often the need for both patients and their family members to reconcile (I'm sorry), forgive (I forgive you, please forgive me), affirm (thank you), and have closure (Goodbye, it's okay for you to go when you need to, we will be okay.) It is also critical to address the spiritual needs of patients and their families in these final days of life. Patients and families are often greatly benefited from a life review individually and together. It is essential that patients are able to examine their legacy and meaning of their life, along with having a peace with a higher God and an afterlife. Any angst of nonexistence or existential suffering must be addressed, as this form of suffering is often the most severe.

As patients enter into the last hours of their life, there tends to be a consistent presentation that providers should recognize and use for patient care and education with the families. Physical signs associated with survival less than 24 hours include

---

Box 5
Physical changes in the last 72 hours of life: central nervous system

Most common

- Withdrawal from others
  - Less communicative, interactions with only a few people
  - The stare
  - The rally: may or may not happen

- Sedation
  - Sleeping much more throughout the day

- Loss of normal circadian rhythms

Less common

- Agitation/paranoia

- Terminal delirium: can be difficult to reverse, with best results in using haloperidol

- Neuroexcitation: myoclonus, sometimes progressing to seizures

---

Box 6
Physical changes in the last 72 hours of life: respiratory and circulatory

Respiratory

- Breathing patterns
  - Cheyne-Stokes
  - Irregularity with pauses increasing over time
- Reflexive accessory muscle usage
  - Chin lift, jaw jerk
  - Shoulder shrug

Circulatory

- Physical signs
  - Third spacing common
  - Mottling of hands, feet, tip of nose, perioral, knees
  - Tachycardia, then terminal bradycardia to asystole
  - Decreasing blood pressure over time
  - Not uncommon for vitals to be fairly normal right up until death

---

- Loss of radial pulse
- Onset of jaw jerk with each breath
- Onset of rattle due to excessive upper airway secretions
- Terminal fever
- Terminal delirium

In terms of providing family education in the last few hours of life, it is beneficial to recognize that family members, as well as sometimes staff, are often poor judges of pain and anxiety in patients. There may also be a lack of understanding concerning hydration and nutrition issues as well as why certain medications are being used or stopped. Addressing these issues may provide significant comfort to the family, while avoiding miscommunication and distress. In addition, discussion on how to best handle the children in the family can also be crucial at this time. Some of these critical family and staff education points are listed in **Box 8.**

Box 7
Physical changes in the last 72 hours of life: genitourinary and gastrointestinal

Genitourinary

- Physical signs
  - Decreased urine output
  - Bladder outlet obstruction
    - Rule out as cause of pain, agitation, or delirium at end of life
    - Not uncommon, especially if patients are on opioids or anticholinergics

Gastrointestinal

- Physical signs
  - Decreased appetite/anorexia
  - Ileus with bloating and nausea/cramping with oral intake
  - Decreased stooling
    - Usually do not aggressively intervene, unless patients are experiencing significant discomfort from distention or impaction

---

Box 8
Critical family/staff education points

Education points

- Teach families to recognize the common physical signs: signposts.
  - It may help prepare for the moment.

- The patients are dying of the underlying disease, not the medicines.

- The right amount of medicine is the amount to be comfortable, no more, no less.

- The ultimate length of the dying process is out of our hands.
  - We only manage its course over its hours to days.

- Do not assume patients cannot hear what loved ones are saying.

- People seem to go on their own time: maybe wait for someone, maybe wait until alone, maybe wait until given permission by loved ones.

- It is common to see and talk to deceased loved ones.

SUMMARY

This article attempts to provide an overview of how integrating quality palliative and end-of-life care into the geriatric assessment can be a tremendous benefit to our older adult patients and their families. Although there are many opportunities to improve the quality of life and function of our older adult patients in the last few years of their life, there are also still a great many general and specific challenges to providing quality palliative and end-of-life care in United States as well as many other countries, as shown in **Box 9**.

Although the quality of palliative and end-of-life care for older adults has improved greatly in recent decades, there is still much that is suboptimal. Many education, communication, coordination of care, organizational, and financial barriers still exist to the ideal provision of palliative and end-of-life care in the US health care system.

Box 9
Challenges to quality palliative and end-of-life care in the United States

General challenges

- There is ambivalence in American culture about death and dying.

- Aging US population is becoming more racially and ethnically diverse.

- Health care providers from diverse backgrounds may have different perspectives.

- Newer and more advanced technological services continually become available and are desired.

- Both physicians and patients may be reluctant to move from cure-directed to comfort-directed care, which may be perceived as giving up.

Specific challenges

- Education, communication, coordination of care, organizational, and financial barriers exist to the ideal use of palliative and end-of-life care in the US health system.

- Clinical expertise in comprehensive palliative and end of life will need to be developed and maintained on a widespread basis.

- Focused and direct reimbursement to physicians for palliative and end-of-life care is needed.

There must be much more clinical expertise in comprehensive palliative care and end of life developed and maintained on a widespread basis for our older adults. In addition, there also must be a greater focus on and more direct reimbursement developed for both physicians and health system providers to provide quality palliative and end-of-life care for the older adult population.

REFERENCES

1. Mack JW, Smith TJ. Reasons why physicians do not have discussions about poor prognosis, why it matters, and what can be improved. J Clin Oncol 2012;30(22): 2715-7.
2. Von Roenn JH, Von Gunten CF. Setting goals to maintain hope. J Clin Oncol 2003; 21(3):570-4.
3. Smith S, Brick A, O'Hara S, et al. Evidence on the cost and cost effectiveness of palliative care: a literature review. Palliat Med 2014;28(2):130-50.
4. NCCN guidelines for supportive care. Available at: http://www.nccn.org/professionals/physician_gls/f_guidelines.asp#survivorship. Accessed July 30, 2016.
5. Goodlin S. Framework for improving care. In: American Academy of Hospice and Palliative Medicine bulletin. Available at: http://www.aahpm.org. Accessed July 30, 2016.
6. Hennessy JE, Lown BA, Landzaat L, et al. Practical issues in palliative and quality-of-life care. J Oncol Pract 2013;9(2):78-80.
7. WHO definition of palliative care. Available at: http://www.who.int/cancer/pallaitive/defination/en. Accessed August 1, 2016.
8. Global atlas of palliative care at the end of life. Worldwide Hospice Palliative Care Alliance and World Health Organization. Available at: http://www.who.int/nmh/Global_Atlas_of_Palliative_Care.pdf. Accessed August 1, 2016.
9. Teno JM, Freedman VA, Kasper JD, et al. Is care for the dying improving in the United States? J Palliat Med 2015;18(8):662-6.
10. Swagerty DL. Integrating palliative care in the nursing home: an interprofessional opportunity. J Am Med Dir Assoc 2014;15(11):863-5.
11. Ghosh A, Dzeng E, Cheng MJ. Interaction of palliative care and primary care. Clin Geriatr Med 2015;31(2):207-18.
12. Weeks JC, Catalano PJ, Cronin A, et al. Patients' expectations about effects of chemotherapy for advanced cancer. N Engl J Med 2013;367(17):1616-25.
13. Smith TJ, Longo DL. Talking to patients about dying. N Engl J Med 2013;368(5): 481.
14. Christakis N. Extent and determinants of error in doctor's prognoses in terminally ill patients: prospective cohort study. BMJ 2000;320(7233):469-72.
15. Evans LR, Boyd EA, Malvar G, et al. Surrogate decision-makers' perspective on discussing prognosis in the face of uncertainty. Am J Respir Crit Care Med 2009; 179(1):48-53.
16. Old J, Swagerty D. Historical perspective; what has changed? Practical guide to palliative care. Lippincott; 2007. p. 10-1.
17. Corr CA. Death in modern society. In: Doyle D, editor. Oxford textbook of medicine. 2nd edition. New York: Oxford University Press; 1998. p. 1-5.
18. Doyle D, et al. Introduction. In: Doyle D, editor. Oxford textbook of medicine. 2nd edition. New York: Oxford University Press; 1998. p. 33.
19. Old J, Swagerty D. The transition from "diagnose and treat" to "palliate" practical guide to palliative care. Lippincott; 2007. p. 8-9.

20. World Health Organization. Cancer pain relief and palliative care. Technical report series 804. Geneva (Switzerland): World Health Organization; 1990.
21. Caring Connections - What is hospice? Available at: http://www.caringinfo.org. Accessed August 2, 2016.
22. Old J, Swagerty D. "How long do I have?" practical guide to palliative care. Lippincott; 2007. p. 89–90.
23. CMS LCD L32015 Hospice determining terminal status. Available at: http://www. nhpco.org/nhpco/ensuring-compliant-hospice-admission-determining-eligibility-prognosis. Accessed August 2, 2016.
24. Old J, Swagerty D. Palliative performance scale. Practical guide to palliative care. Lippincott; 2007. p. 95–6.

Rapid Geriatric Assessment
Secondary Prevention to Stop Age-Associated Disability

John E. Morley, MB, BCh[a,b],*

KEYWORDS

- Rapid Geriatric Assessment • Frailty • Sarcopenia • Anorexia
- Cognition and advanced directives • Early intervention

KEY POINTS

- The Rapid Geriatric Assessment measures frailty, sarcopenia, anorexia, cognition, and advanced directives.
- The Rapid Geriatric Assessment is a screen for primary care physicians to be able to detect geriatric syndromes.
- Early intervention when geriatric syndromes are recognized can decrease disability, hospitalization, and mortality.

With the rapid increase in the aging population over the first half of this century and a paucity of geriatricians worldwide, there is a major need to enhance the ability of primary care physicians and advance practice nurses to recognize and manage geriatric syndromes.[1–3] Numerous studies have shown that geriatric evaluation and management reduces disability, hospitalization, and nursing home placement and delays death.[4–6] In the past decade it has been widely recognized that certain geriatric syndromes, frailty, sarcopenia, anorexia of aging, and cognitive impairment, are the major causes of poor outcomes in older persons.[7–10] To increase the awareness and management of these geriatric giants at Saint Louis University, the author and colleagues have developed the Rapid Geriatric Assessment (RGA) to screen for geriatric syndromes and provide a computer-assisted management system for primary care health professionals[11] (**Fig. 1**).

[a] Division of Geriatric Medicine, Saint Louis University School of Medicine, 1402 South Grand Boulevard, M238, St Louis, MO 63104, USA; [b] Division of Endocrinology, Saint Louis University School of Medicine, 1402 South Grand Boulevard, M238, St Louis, MO 63104, USA
* Division of Geriatric Medicine, Saint Louis University School of Medicine, 1402 South Grand Boulevard, M238, St Louis, MO 63104.
E-mail address: morley@slu.edu

Clin Geriatr Med 33 (2017) 431–440
http://dx.doi.org/10.1016/j.cger.2017.03.006
0749-0690/17/© 2017 Elsevier Inc. All rights reserved.

Saint Louis University
Rapid Geriatric Assessment

The Simple "FRAIL" Questionnaire Screening Tool
(3 or greater = frailty; 1 or 2 = prefrail)

Fatigue: Are you fatigued?
Resistance: Cannot walk up one flight of stairs?
Aerobic: Cannot walk one block?
Illnesses: Do you have more than 5 illnesses?
Loss of weight: Have you lost more than 5% of your weight
in the last 6 mo?

From Morley JE, Vellas B, Abellan van Kan G, et al. J Am Med Dir Assoc
2013;14:392-397.

Table I: SARC-F Screen for Sarcopenia

Component	Question	Scoring
Strength	How much difficulty do you have in lifting and carrying 10 pounds?	None = 0 Some = 1 A lot or unable = 2
Assistance in walking	How much difficulty do you have walking across a room?	None = 0 Some = 1 A lot, use aids, or unable = 2
Rise from a chair	How much difficulty do you have transferring from a chair or bed?	None = 0 Some = 1 A lot or unable without help = 2
Climb stairs	How much difficulty do you have climbing a flight of ten stairs?	None = 0 Some = 1 A lot or unable = 2
Falls	How many times have you fallen in the last year?	None = 0 1–3 falls = 1 4 or more falls = 2

From Malmstrom TK, Morley JE. J Frailty and Aging 2013;2:55-6.

SNAQ (Simplified Nutritional Assessment Questionnaire)

My appetite is
a. very poor
b. poor
c. average
d. good
e. very good

Food tastes
a. very bad
b. bad
c. average
d. good
e. very good

When I eat
a. I feel full after eating only a few mouthfuls
b. I feel full after eating about a third of a meal
c. I feel full after eating over half a meal
d. I feel full after eating most of the meal
e. I hardly ever feel full

Normally I eat
a. less than one meal a day
b. one meal a day
c. two meals a day
d. three meals a day
e. more than three meals a day

From Wilson et al. Am J Clin Nutr 2005;82:1074-81.

Rapid Cognitive Screen (RCS)

1. **Please remember these five objects. I will ask you what they are later.** [Read each object to patient using approx. 1 second intervals.]
Apple   Pen   Tie   House   Car
2. [Give patient pencil and the blank sheet with clock face.] **This is a clock face. Please put in the hour markers and the time at ten minutes to eleven o'clock.** [2 pts/hr markers ok; 2 pts/time correct]
3. **What were the five objects I asked you to remember?** [1 pt/ea]
4. **I'm going to tell you a story. Please listen carefully because afterwards, I'm going to ask you about it.**

Jill was a very successful stockbroker. She made a lot of money on the stock market. She then met Jack, a devastatingly handsome man. She married him and had three children. They lived in Chicago. She then stopped work and stayed at home to bring up her children. When they were teenagers, she went back to work. She and Jack lived happily ever after.
What state did she live in? [1 pt]

From Malmstrom TK, Voss VB, Cruz-Oliver DM et al.
J Nutr Health Aging 2015;19:741-744.

Miscellaneous
Are you constipated? Y/N
Do you have worrisome incontinence? Y/N
Do you have an advanced directive? Y/N

Fig. 1. Saint Louis University RGA. There is no copyright on these screening tools and they may be incorporated into the Electronic Health Record without permission and at no cost.

THE PHYSICAL FRAILTY PHENOTYPE

Fried and her colleagues[12] developed a screening test for physical frailty consisting of self-reported exhaustion, weakness (grip strength), slow walking speed, and low physical activity. Numerous studies have subsequently validated this as a screening test.[13–15] Subsequently, the FRAIL, a simple screening test[16] consisting of 5 questions, has been developed:

F: Are you fatigued?
R (resistance): Are you not able to walk up a flight of stairs?
A (aerobic): Can you not walk a block (200 m)?
I: Do you have more than 5 illnesses?
L: Have you lost 5% of your weight in the last 6 months?

One or 2 positive questions is categorized as prefrail, and 3 or more is frail.
This questionnaire's predictive value has been validated in Australia,[17–20] Asia,[21–23] Europe,[24,25] the United States,[26–28] and Mexico.[29] It has been shown to have similar sensitivity and specificity to the Fried (Cardiovascular Health Study) physical frailty phenotype and the Rockwood multi-morbidity scale.[23,28] In nursing homes, a variant of this scale (FRAIL-NH), has been shown to be equally predictive of poor outcomes.[30,31]

Early recognition of frailty is important as a combination of exercise, protein supplementation, and/or vitamin D has been demonstrated to reverse the frailty characteristics and decrease disability and hospitalization.[32–36]

The RGA computer-assisted management system not only recommends the exercise and nutrition program but if the person answers positive for fatigue suggests that person be investigated for sleep apnea,[37] hypotension including postural hypotension,[38] depression,[39] hypothyroidism,[40] vitamin B12 deficiency,[41] and anemia.[42] The health professional is prompted to consider polypharmacy as a cause if the person has more than 5 illnesses,[43–46] with an emphasis on medications that are inappropriate for older persons.[38] If the person has weight loss, the physician is asked to check for reversible causes using the MEALS-ON-WHEELS mnemonic[47,48]:

M = medications
E = emotional (depression)
A = elder ABUSE, alcoholism
L = late-life paranoia
S = swallowing disorders

O = oral conditions
N = nosocomial infections, for example, tuberculosis, *Helicobacter pylori*

W = wandering and other dementia-related behaviors
H = hyperthyroidism, hypertension, (pheochromocytoma), hypercalcemia, and Addison disease
E = enteral problems (celiac disease, pancreatic disease)
E = eating problems
L = low cholesterol, low salt, therapeutic diets
S = stones (cholecystitis)

SARCOPENIA

Sarcopenia has been defined as decreased muscle function (walking speed or 6-minute walk distance) or strength (grip strength) associated with a low muscle mass.[49–53] These values need to be adjusted for different ethnicity. The definitions have been validated.[54–58] All of these definitions require measurement of muscle mass and physical measurements of strength. There is now an *International Classification of Diseases, Tenth Revision, Clinical Modification* code for sarcopenia that makes it a billable diagnosis.

SARC-F is a simple questionnaire that identified people with sarcopenia.[8,59,60] It has been validated in Asia,[61–63] the United States,[27,64] and Europe. About one-third of people with sarcopenia are not frail, and a third of people who are frail are not sarcopenic.[65]

For SARC-F–positive individuals, the computer-assisted management program recommends resistance exercise,[35,66–68] leucine-enriched essential amino acid supplementation,[69,70] and 1000 IU of vitamin D daily.[71]

SIMPLIFIED NUTRITIONAL ASSESSMENT QUESTIONNAIRE

Weight loss is a major indicator of risk for hospitalization, institutionalization, and death in older persons.[72] The anorexia of aging both as a physiologic and pathologic condition is now well recognized as a risk factor for weight loss, sarcopenia,[73] and cachexia.[74] The Simplified Nutritional Assessment Questionnaire has been validated as a useful predictor of future weight loss in Japan,[75] Europe,[76] and the United States.[77]

The computer-assisted management program recommends liquid caloric supplementation[78] and to look for treatable causes as described in the weight loss section of frailty.

RAPID COGNITIVE SCREEN

Early recognition of cognitive impairment is important, as it may be treatable. In one study, approximately half of the persons with mild cognitive impairment (MCI) who received a geriatric assessment had normal cognition 6 years later.[79] Reversible causes of MCI and dementia are easily identified using the DEMENTIAS mnemonic[80]:

D = drugs (anticholinergic)[81,82]
E = emotional (depression)
M = metabolic (hypothyroid, diabetes)
E = eyes and ears impairment
N = normal pressure hydrocephalus (dementia, balance problems, incontinence)
T = tumors and other space-occupying lesions
I = infections
A = atrial fibrillation, alcoholism
S = sleep apnea[83]

Other reasons for early recognition of cognitive impairment are

- It allows the physician to recognize the need for written instructions and in some cases to have a carer present.
- It provides recognition that the person may not be able to drive or have the ability to manage his or her own medicines.
- It allows time to develop advance directives.[84]
- There is evidence that a Mediterranean diet, extra virgin olive oil, exercise, and intellectual games in combination may slow cognitive decline.[85–91]
- In persons with a moderate cognitive deficit, cognitive stimulation therapy improves memory.

It is now well established that both the Montreal Cognitive Assessment[92] and the Saint Louis University Mental Status (SLUMS) examination[93,94] are superior to the Mini-Mental State Examination for recognizing MCI. The SLUMS is available in more than 30 languages (aging.slu.edu). The Rapid Cognitive Screen (RCS) was developed from the SLUMS using the 3 questions with best sensitivity and specificity. The RCS takes 2.5 minutes to conduct. It is better than the Mini-Cog.[95]

ADVANCE DIRECTIVES

There are major advantages to the person and the health system for older persons to have developed advanced directives.[96] The RGA includes a question on advance directives.

SUMMARY

The RGA has been developed to provide a simple, computer-assisted system for recognition and management of geriatric syndromes. Woo and colleagues,[21] using the FRAIL and SARC-F with a different cognitive screen, showed that this approach has similar ability to the comprehensive geriatric assessment to recognize geriatric syndromes. The author and colleagues' experience in Missouri, as part of their Geriatric Workforce Enhancement Program grant, is that it is easily used by office staff in physicians' offices. It can be used as a major component of the Medicare annual wellness visit.[97]

REFERENCES

1. Fougere B, Morley JE, Decavel F, et al. Development and implementation of the advanced practice nurse worldwide with an interest in geriatric care. J Am Med Dir Assoc 2016;17(9):782–8.
2. Yang M, Chang CH, Carmichael D, et al. Who is providing the predominant care for older adults with dementia? J Am Med Dir Assoc 2016;17(9):802–6.
3. Morley JE. Aging successfully: the key to aging in place. J Am Med Dir Assoc 2015;18:1005–7.
4. Rubenstein LZ. Evolving models of comprehensive geriatric assessment. J Am Med Dir Assoc 2015;16:446–7.
5. Huss A, Stuck AE, Rubenstein LZ, et al. Multidimensional preventive home visit programs for community-dwelling older adults: a systematic review and meta-analysis of randomized controlled trials. J Gerontol A Biol Sci Med Sci 2008;63:298–307.
6. Stuck AE, Siu AL, Wieland GD, et al. Comprehensive geriatric assessment: a meta-analysis of controlled trials. Lancet 1993;342:1031–6.
7. Morley JE. Developing novel therapeutic approaches to frailty. Curr Pharm Des 2009;15:3384–95.
8. Morley JE, Cao L. Rapid screening for sarcopenia. J Cachexia Sarcopenia Muscle 2015;6:312–4.
9. Morley JE. Weight loss in older persons: new therapeutic approaches. Curr Pharm Des 2007;13:3637–47.
10. Morley JE, Morris JC, Berg-Weger M, et al. Brain health: the importance of recognizing cognitive impairment: an IAGG consensus conference. J Am Med Dir Assoc 2015;16:731–9.
11. Morley JE, Adams EV. Rapid geriatric assessment. J Am Med Dir Assoc 2015;16:808–12.
12. Fried LP, Tangen CM, Walston J, et al. Frailty in older adults: evidence for a phenotype. J Gerontol A Biol Sci Med Sci 2001;56:M146–56.
13. Fried LP, Ferrucci L, Darer J, et al. Untangling the concepts of disability, frailty, and comorbidity: implications for improved targeting and care. J Gerontol A Biol Sci Med Sci 2004;59:255–63.
14. Theou O, Walston J, Rockwood K. Operationalizing frailty using the frailty phenotype and deficit accumulation approaches. Interdiscip Top Gerontol Geriatr 2015;41:66–73.
15. Morley JE, Vellas B, van Kan GA, et al. Frailty consensus: a call to action. J Am Med Dir Assoc 2013;14:392–7.
16. Abellan van Kan G, Rolland Y, Bergman H, et al. The I.A.N.A. task force on frailty assessment of older people in clinical practice. J Nutr Health Aging 2008;12:29–37.
17. Hyde Z, Flicker L, Smith K, et al. Prevalence and incidence of frailty in Aboriginal Australians, and associations with mortality and disability. Maturitas 2016;87:89–94.
18. Gardiner PA, Mishra GD, Dobson AJ. Validity and responsiveness of the FRAIL scale in a longitudinal cohort study of older Australian women. J Am Med Dir Assoc 2015;16:781–3.
19. Hyde Z, Flicker L, Dobson A. Validation of the frail scale in a cohort of older Australian women. J Am Geriatr Soc 2012;60:171–3.
20. Hyde Z, Flicker L, Almeida OP, et al. Low free testosterone predicts frailty in older men: the health in men study. J Clin Endocrinol Metab 2010;95:3165–72.

21. Woo J, Yu R, Wong M, et al. Frailty screening in the community using the FRAIL scale. J Am Med Dir Assoc 2015;16:412–9.
22. Li Y, Zou Y, Wang S, et al. A pilot study of the FRAIL scale on predicting outcomes in Chinese elderly people with type 2 diabetes. J Am Med Dir Assoc 2015;16:714.e-12.
23. Woo J, Leung J, Morley JE. Comparison of frailty indicators based on clinical phenotype and the multiple deficit approach in predicting mortality and physical limitation. J Am Geriatr Soc 2012;60:1478–86.
24. Theou O, Brothers TD, Mitnitski A, et al. Operationalization of frailty using eight commonly used scales and comparison of their ability to predict all-cause mortality. J Am Geriatr Soc 2013;61:1537–51.
25. Ravindrarajah R, Lee DM, Pye SR, et al. The ability of three different models of frailty to predict all-cause mortality: results from the European Male Aging Study (EMAS). Arch Gerontol Geriatr 2013;57:360–8.
26. Morley JE, Malmstrom TK, Miller DK. A simple frailty questionnaire (FRAIL) predicts outcomes in middle aged African Americans. J Nutr Health Aging 2012;16:601–8.
27. Liccini A, Malmstrom TK. Frailty and sarcopenia as predictors of adverse health outcomes in persons with diabetes mellitus. J Am Med Dir Assoc 2016;17:846–51.
28. Malmstrom TK, Miller DK, Morley JE. A comparison of four frailty models. J Am Geriatr Soc 2014;62:721–6.
29. Diaz de Leon Gonzalez E, Guiterrez Hermosillo H, Martinez Beltran JA, et al. Validation of the frail scale in Mexican elderly: results from the Mexican Health and Aging Study. Aging Clin Exp Res 2015;28(5):901–8.
30. Kaehr EW, Pape LC, Malmstrom TK, et al. FRAIL-NH predicts outcomes in long term care. J Nutr Health Aging 2016;20:192–8.
31. Luo H, Lum TY, Wong GH, et al. Predicting adverse health outcomes in nursing homes: a 9-year longitudinal study and development of the FRAIL-minimum data set (MS) quick screening tool. J Am Med Dir Assoc 2015;16:1042–7.
32. Tarazona-Santabalbina JF, Gomez-Cabrera MC, Perez-Ros P, et al. A multicomponent exercise intervention that reverses frailty and improves cognition, emotion, and social networking in the community-dwelling frail elderly: a randomized clinical trial. J Am Med Dir Assoc 2016;17:426–33.
33. Abizanda P, Lopez MD, Garcia VP, et al. Effects of an oral nutritional supplementation plus physical exercise intervention on the physical function, nutritional status, and quality of life in frail institutionalized older adults: the ACTIVNES study. J Am Med Dir Assoc 2015;16:439.e-16.
34. Tp Ng, Feng L, Nyunt MS, et al. Nutritional, physical, cognitive, and combination interventions and frailty reversal among older adults: a randomized controlled trial. Am J Med 2015;128:1225–36.e1.
35. Singh NA, Quine S, Clemson LM, et al. Effects of high-intensity progressive resistance training and targeted multidisciplinary treatment of frailty on mortality and nursing home admissions after hip fracture: a randomized controlled trial. J Am Med Dir Assoc 2012;13:24–30.
36. Theou O, Stathokostas L, Roland KP, et al. The effectiveness of exercise interventions for the management of frailty: a systematic review. J Aging Res 2011;2011:569194.
37. Morley JE. Sleep and the nursing home. J Am Med Dir Assoc 2015;16:539–43.
38. Morley JE. Inappropriate drug prescribing and polypharmacy are major causes of poor outcomes in long-term care. J Am Med Dir Assoc 2014;15:780–2.

39. Thakur M, Blazer DG. Depression in long-term care. J Am Med Dir Assoc 2008;9: 82–7.
40. Dominguez LJ, Bevilacqua M, Dibella G, et al. Diagnosing and managing thyroid disease in the nursing home. J Am Med Dir Assoc 2008;9:9–17.
41. Iwanczyk L, Weintraub NT, Rubenstein LZ. Orthostatic hypotension in the nursing home setting. J Am Med Dir Assoc 2006;7:163–7.
42. Morley JE. Anemia in the nursing homes: a complex issue. J Am Med Dir Assoc 2012;13:191–4.
43. Moulis F, Moulis G, Balardy L, et al. Searching for a polypharmacy threshold associated with frailty. J Am Med Dir Assoc 2015;16:259–61.
44. Moulis F, Moulis G, Balardy L, et al. Exposure to atropinic drugs and frailty status. J Am Med Dir Assoc 2015;16:253–7.
45. Rolland Y, Morley JE. Editorial: frailty and polypharmacy. J Nutr Health Aging 2016;20:645–6.
46. Little MO, Morley A. Reducing polypharmacy: evidence from a simple quality improvement initiative. J Am Med Dir Assoc 2013;14:152–6.
47. Morley JE. Anorexia of aging: a true geriatric syndrome. J Nutr Health Aging 2012;16:422–5.
48. Morley JE. Anorexia, weight loss, and frailty. J Am Med Dir Assoc 2010;11:225–8.
49. Cruz-Jentoft AJ, Baeyens JP, Bauer JM, et al. Sarcopenia: European consensus on definition and diagnosis: report of the European Working Group on Sarcopenia in Older People. Age Ageing 2010;39:412–23.
50. Dam TT, Peters KW, Fragala M, et al. An evidence-based comparison of operational criteria for the presence of sarcopenia. J Gerontol A Biol Sci 2014;69: 584–90.
51. Morley JE, Abbatecola AM, Argiles JM, et al, Society on Sarcopenia, Cachexia and Wasting Disorders Trialist Workshop. Sarcopenia with limited mobility: an international consensus. J Am Med Dir Assoc 2011;12:403–9.
52. Fielding RA, Vellas B, Evans WJ, et al. Sarcopenia: an undiagnosed condition in older adults. Current consensus definition: prevalence, etiology, and consequences. International Working Group on Sarcopenia. J Am Med Dir Assoc 2011;12:249–56.
53. Chen LK, Liu LK, Woo J, et al. Sarcopenia in Asia: consensus report of the Asian Working Group for Sarcopenia. J Am Med Dir Assoc 2014;15:95–101.
54. Lee WJ, Liu LK, Peng LN, et al, ILAS Research Group. Comparisons of sarcopenia defined by IWGS and EWGSOP criteria among older people: results from the I-Lan longitudinal aging study. J Am Med Dir Assoc 2013;14:528.e1–7.
55. Kim YP, Kim S, John JY, et al. Effect of interaction between dynapenic component of the European working group on sarcopenia in older people, sarcopenia criteria and obesity on activities of daily living in the elderly. J Am Med Dir Assoc 2014; 15:371.e1–5.
56. Malmstrom TK, Miller DK, Herning MM, et al. Low appendicular skeletal muscle mass (ASM) with limited mobility and poor health outcomes in middle-aged African Americans. J Cachexia Sarcopenia Muscle 2013;4:179–86.
57. Woo J, Leung J, Morley JE. Defining sarcopenia in terms of incident adverse outcomes. J Am Med Dir Assoc 2015;16:247–52.
58. Dupuy C, Lauwers-Cances V, Guyonnet S, et al. Searching for a relevant definition of sarcopenia: results from the cross-sectional EPIDOS study. J Cachexia Sarcopenia Muscle 2015;6:144–54.
59. Morley JE, Malmstrom TK. Can sarcopenia be diagnosed without measurements? Eur Geriatr Med 2014;5:291–3.

60. Morley JE, Anker SD, von Haehling S. Prevalence, incidence, and clinical impact of sarcopenia: facts, numbers, and epidemiology – update 2014. J Cachexia Sarcopenia Muscle 2014;5:253–9.

61. Woo J, Leung J, Morley JE. Validating the SARC-F: a suitable community screening tool for sarcopenia? J Am Med Dir Assoc 2014;15:630–4.

62. Cao L, Chen S, Zou C, et al. A pilot study of the SARC-F scale on screening sarcopenia and physical disability in the Chinese older people. J Nutr Health Aging 2014;18:277–83.

63. Wu T-Y, Liaw C-K, Chen F-C, et al. Sarcopenia diagnosed with SARC-F questionnaire is associated with quality of life and four-year-mortality. J Am Med Dir Assoc 2016;17:1129–35.

64. Malmstrom TM, Miller DK, Simonsick EM, et al. SARC-F: a symptom score to predict persons with sarcopenia at risk for poor functional outcomes. J Cachexia Sarcopenia Muscle 2016;7:28–36.

65. Mijnarends DM, Schols JM, Meijers JM, et al. Instruments to assess sarcopenia and physical frailty in older people living in a community (care) setting: similarities and discrepancies. J Am Med Dir Assoc 2015;16:301–8.

66. Kim HK, Suzuki T, Saito K, et al. Effects of exercise and amino acid supplementation on body composition and physical function in community-dwelling elderly Japanese sarcopenic women: a randomized controlled trial. J Am Geriatr Soc 2012;60:16–23.

67. Yamada M, Nishiguchi S, Fukutani N, et al. Mail-based intervention for sarcopenia prevention increased anabolic hormone and skeletal muscle mass in community-dwelling Japanese older adults: the INE (Intervention by Nutrition and Exercise) study. J Am Med Dir Assoc 2015;16:654–60.

68. Churchward-Venne TA, Tieland M, Verdijk LB, et al. There are no nonresponders to resistance-type exercise training in older men and women. J Am Med Dir Assoc 2015;16:400–11.

69. Bauer JM, Verlaan S, Bautmans I, et al. Effects of vitamin D and leucine-enriched whey protein nutritional supplement on measures of sarcopenia in older adults, the PROVIDE study: a randomized, double-blind, placebo-controlled trial. J Am Med Dir Assoc 2015;16:740–7.

70. Bauer J, Biolo G, Cederholm T, et al. Evidence-based recommendations for optimal dietary protein intake in older people: a position paper from the PROT-AGE study group. J Am Med Dir Assoc 2013;14:542–59.

71. Beaudart C, Buckinx F, Rabenda V, et al. The effects of vitamin D on skeletal muscle strength, muscle mass, and muscle power: a systematic review and meta-analysis of randomized controlled trials. J Clin Endocrinol Metab 2014;99:4336–45.

72. Martone AM, Onder G, Vetrano DL, et al. Anorexia of aging: a modifiable risk factor for frailty. Nutrients 2013;5:4126–33.

73. Cheng Q, Zhu X, Zhang X, et al. A cross-sectional study of loss of muscle mass corresponding to sarcopenia in healthy Chinese men and women: reference values, prevalence, and association with bone mass. J Bone Miner Metab 2014;32:78–88.

74. Anker SD, Morley JE. Cachexia: a nutritional syndrome? J Cachexia Sarcopenia Muscle 2015;6:269–71.

75. Nakatsu N, Sawa R, Misu S, et al. Reliability and validity of the Japanese version of the simplified nutritional appetite questionnaire in community-dwelling older adults. Geriatr Gerontol Int 2015;15:1264–9.

76. Rolland Y, Perrin A, Gardette V, et al. Screening older people at risk of malnutrition or malnourished using the Simplified Nutritional Appetite Questionnaire (SNAQ): a comparison with the mini-nutritional assessment (MNA) tool. J Am Med Dir Assoc 2012;13:31–4.

77. Wilson MM, Thomas DR, Rubenstein LZ, et al. Appetite assessment: simple appetite questionnaire predicts weight loss in community-dwelling adults and nursing home residents. Am J Clin Nutr 2005;82:1074–81.

78. Wilson MM, Purushothaman R, Morley JE. Effect of liquid dietary supplements on energy intake in the elderly. Am J Clin Nutr 2002;75:944–7.

79. Cruz-Oliver DM, Malmstrom TK, Roegner M, et al. Cognitive deficit reversal as shown by changes in the Veterans Affairs Saint Louis University mental status (SLUMS) examination scores 7.5 years later. J Am Med Dir Assoc 2014;15: 687.e5-10.

80. Morley JE. Mild cognitive impairment – a treatable condition. J Am Med Dir Assoc 2014;15:1–5.

81. Bishara D, Harwood D, Sauer J, et al. Anticholinergic effect on cognition (AEC) of drugs commonly used in older people. Int J Geriatr Psychiatry 2016. [Epub ahead of print].

82. Lowry E, Woodman RJ, Soiza R, et al. Associations between the anticholinergic risk scale score and physical function: potential implications for adverse outcomes in older hospitalized patients. J Am Med Dir Assoc 2011;12:565–72.

83. Buratti L, Luzzi S, Petrelli C, et al. Obstructive sleep apnea syndrome: an emerging risk factor for dementia. CNS Neurol Disord Drug Targets 2016;15(6): 678–82.

84. Abele P, Morley JE. Advance directives: the key to a good death? J Am Med Dir Assoc 2016;17:279–83.

85. Shah R. The role of nutrition and diet in Alzheimer disease: a systematic review. J Am Med Dir Assoc 2013;14:398–402.

86. Lee AT, Richards M, Chan WC, et al. Intensity and types of physical exercise in relation to dementia risk reduction in community-living older adults. J Am Med Dir Assoc 2015;16:899.e1–7.

87. Brett L, Traynor V, Stapley P. Effects of physical exercise on health and well-being of individuals living with a dementia in nursing homes: a systematic review. J Am Med Dir Assoc 2016;17:104–16.

88. Farr SA, Price TO, Dominguez LJ, et al. Extra virgin olive oil improves learning and memory in SAMP8 mice. J Alzheimers Dis 2012;28:81–92.

89. Martinez-Lapiscina EH, Clavero P, Toledo E, et al. Virgin olive oil supplementation and long-term cognition: the PREDIMED-NAVARRA randomized, trial. J Nutr Health Aging 2013;17:544–52.

90. D'Amico F, Rehill A, Knapp M, et al. Maintenance cognitive stimulation therapy: an economic evaluation within a randomized controlled trial. J Am Med Dir Assoc 2015;16:63–70.

91. Ngandu T, Lehtisalo J, Solomon A, et al. A 2 year multidomain intervention of diet, exercise, cognitive training, and vascular risk monitoring versus control to prevent cognitive decline in at-risk elderly people (FINGER): a randomised controlled trial. Lancet 2015;385:2255–63.

92. Shaik MA, Chan QL, Xu J, et al. Risk factors of cognitive impairment and brief cognitive tests to predict cognitive performance determined by a formal neuropsychological evaluation of primary health care patients. J Am Med Dir Assoc 2016;17:343–7.

93. Cruz-Oliver DM, Malmstrom TK, Allen CM, et al. The Veterans Affairs Saint Louis University mental status exam (SLUMS exam) and the mini-mental status exam as predictors of mortality and institutionalization. J Nutr Health Aging 2012;16: 636–41.
94. Tariq SH, Tumosa N, Chibnall JT, et al. Comparison of the Saint Louis University mental status examination and the mini-mental state examination for detecting dementia and mild neurocognitive disorder—a pilot study. Am J Geriatr Psychiatry 2006;14:900–10.
95. Malmstrom TK, Voss VB, Cruz-Oliver DM, et al. The rapid cognitive screen (RCS): a point-of-care screening for dementia and mild cognitive impairment. J Nutr Health Aging 2015;19:741–4.
96. Schoene-Seifert B, Uerpmann AL, Gerb J, et al. Advance (Meta-) directives for patients with dementia who appear content: learning from a nationwide survey. J Am Med Dir Assoc 2016;17:294–9.
97. Morley JE, Abele P. The Medicare annual wellness visit in nursing homes. J Am Med Dir Assoc 2016;17:567–9.

Index

Note: Page numbers of articles titles are in **boldface** type.

Clin Geriatr Med 33 (2017) 441–446
http://dx.doi.org/10.1016/S0749-0690(17)30046-0
0749-0690/17

geriatric.theclinics.com

Moving?

Make sure your subscription moves with you!

To notify us of your new address, find your **Clinics Account Number** (located on your mailing label above your name), and contact customer service at:

Email: journalscustomerservice-usa@elsevier.com

800-654-2452 (subscribers in the U.S. & Canada)
314-447-8871 (subscribers outside of the U.S. & Canada)

Fax number: 314-447-8029

Elsevier Health Sciences Division
Subscription Customer Service
3251 Riverport Lane
Maryland Heights, MO 63043

Printed and bound by CPI Group (UK) Ltd, Croydon, CR0 4YY

03/10/2024

01040495-0012